The portable studio
Art therapy and political conflict:
initiatives in former Yugoslavia and
KwaZulu–Natal, South Africa

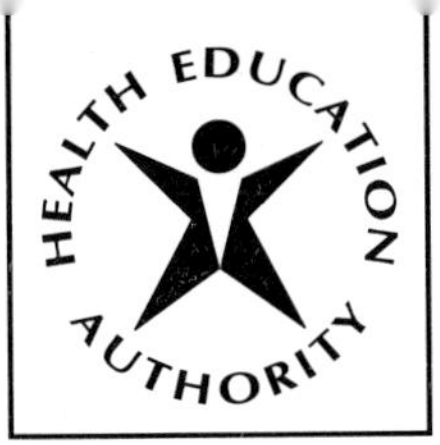

The portable studio
Art therapy and political conflict:

initiatives in former Yugoslavia and KwaZulu–Natal, South Africa

Debra Kalmanowitz and Bobby Lloyd

ISBN 0 7521 0857 3

Contents

Note from the Health Education Authority

'Mental health is the emotional and spiritual resilience which enables us to enjoy life and to survive pain, disappointment and sadness. It is a positive sense of wellbeing and an underlying belief in our own, and others', dignity and worth' (Health Education Authority, 1997)

This publication is one of a wide range of initiatives supported by the Health Education Authority, on behalf of the Department of Health, as part of the World Mental Health Day Campaign. The Campaign aims to increase understanding of the importance of mental health and wellbeing, to reduce the stigma surrounding mental health issues and to provide support and resources for those working to promote mental health across all sectors. Many agencies have a role to play in promoting mental health. The Campaign brings together mental health service users, voluntary agencies, health authorities and local authorities and also aims to highlight opportunities for mental health promotion at all levels – in education, in the workplace, in institutions, families and the community.

Much has been learned in recent years about the benefits of art therapy as part of a healing process for people who have experienced pain, loss and trauma. The projects described in this pioneering book were developed to address the psychological effects of political conflict. However, the learning drawn from the initiatives in the former Yugoslavia and South Africa will be of value to a wide range of professionals working with individuals and communities who have suffered trauma. Art therapy provides a language for exploring and expressing experiences which may be difficult or impossible to put into words. It can be used with children and adults of all ages and in many different settings, including schools, hospitals, prisons and community centres.

This book provides practical information on establishing art therapy initiatives, as well as a literature review and detailed bibliography to assist further research in this area. We very much welcome its publication as a new and valuable contribution to increasing understanding of the role of art therapy in promoting mental health.

Dr Lynne Friedli
Health Education Authority

Foreword

by Diane Waller

This book gives an account of two pilot art therapy projects and an art therapy training workshop, fully describing the context in which the work took place. These practical, informative and very moving accounts include detail in a way which will enable the material to be applied in a broader context. The projects have given rise to two working models for establishing art therapy in the context of political conflict: the first for an art therapy service for children and adults, the second for art therapy workshops for local professionals and carers.

Although the authors have professed that this is not a definitive work, it is my belief that the useful, practical considerations and honest account of obstacles and ways forward make this a highly comprehensive study on the subject and an invaluable document for anyone wishing to work in such a demanding field.

It will be useful to anyone engaged in education working in the field of mental health, in art therapy and other creative arts therapies, for those considering carrying out their own research and for aid workers and organisations who use art in this context.

Readers of this book will be grateful that Debra Kalmanowitz and Bobby Lloyd have persisted in their effort to present this material. It is a timely piece of work in view of the need to offer support and conduct research when faced with devastating psychological effects of political conflict.

Dr Diane Waller
Head of the Art Psychotherapy Unit
Goldsmiths' College
University of London

Foreword

by Shankarnarayan Srinath

'Upon the blackboard of my pillowed eyes
I saw a circle drawn in thick white chalk,
And this was a hole and in this hole, deep down,
I saw my father lying in his coffin, and I
felt nothing.'
Delmore Schwartz in *The Brother Poem*

'Survivorship', Bruno Bettelheim says, 'has two closely related but separate issues. First is the original trauma. Second, there are the lifelong after-effects of such a trauma which seems to require very special forms of mastery if one is not to succumb to them'. Massive traumatic experiences disturb a person's perception of the world. The sense of inner security is shaken and there is often a loss of basic trust. The person is gripped by a nameless dread with confusing feelings of despair, sadness, rage and aggression. Deeply upsetting memories may return to haunt the person again and again. These experiences also evoke moral pain, insistent questions about the meaning of life and guilt for having survived the trauma while others may have perished. Freud, in *Beyond the Pleasure Principle* (Standard edition XVIII), observes that the recurrent nightmares of soldiers suffering from battle neurosis are an attempt by the unconscious mind to overcome the trauma. He suggests that children's play in the wake of a loss may have a similar creative function to help them master the situation.

Therapies are creative attempts to help the survivors make sense of their experience and rebuild their lives. This imposes an enormous and painful burden on them: they must think the unthinkable and mourn the destruction of their world. Survivors so often have difficulty in expressing their intense feelings and they may unconsciously put into action what cannot be put into words and make others feel what they cannot feel themselves. This is all the more so with children for whom the experience is more perplexing and frightening. Therapies based on creative arts such as art therapy help to express and restore symbolically the unspeakable horror of their experience. Creativity confirms the individuals and helps them fathom their nightmares on their own terms.

This book by Debra Kalmanowitz and Bobby Lloyd, both registered art therapists, is about art therapy in the context of war and political conflict. Their work sensitively highlights the therapeutic use of art at these times. The models they propose here, although set in art therapy, deserve a wider reception. They are applicable not only in areas of conflict, but also in this country by professionals working with survivors of trauma. Their work complements the trauma work done by other disciplines and organisations such as the Medical Foundation for the Victims of Torture and the Tavistock Clinic.

Dr Shankarnarayan Srinath
Psychiatrist, Trauma Clinic
Tavistock and Portman Clinic, London

The authors

Debra Kalmanowitz trained in both Israel and the US, and holds a Master's Degree in Expressive Arts Therapy from Lesley College, Cambridge, Massachusetts, USA. She formerly studied Sociology and Anthropology at Hebrew University, Jerusalem, Israel. Debra has worked as an arts therapist in various settings in Israel, Canada, USA and the UK, with both adults and children. Her recent work in London has included working with young offenders at a prison near Heathrow, and at an East London hospice with cancer patients. As well as continuing to develop her own art work, she is at present working in a North London primary school, primarily with refugee children.

Bobby Lloyd trained at Goldsmiths' College, London University, and holds a post-graduate diploma in Art Therapy. She formerly studied Fine Art at Oxford University, the Glasgow School of Art, Scotland and Chicago, USA. As well as exhibiting her own work on a regular basis, her work has included several years as an artist and art therapist at a Central London homeless unit. As the art therapist in the Child and Family Department of a clinic in West London, she hopes to develop a refugee component within the service.

Together they established and co-ordinate the *Art Therapy Initiative* and are regular co-facilitators of art therapy workshops, seminar discussion groups and direct art therapy work with refugee families in London.

Acknowledgements

We would like to express our tremendous gratitude to the individuals we met in Bosnia, Croatia and Slovenia who offered their hospitality. Special thanks to Alma and Ermin in East Mostar and Misha and Jasna in Sarajevo, Bosnia who so generously invited us to stay in their homes and to the individuals in the two refugee centres in which we stayed – Prvic and Hrastnik – with whom we spent many hours drinking coffee, talking and painting. Through them, we were able to better understand and gain insights into this context of war as far as was possible.

We would like to acknowledge the invaluable contributions of Dr Diane Waller, President of the British Association of Art Therapists (BAAT), for the extended periods of supervision offered to us in her own time, Michael Anderson, community artist, for his important work on the pilot art therapy project at Hrastnik, and all those individuals and organisations who generously contributed money to enable the visits and on-site work to take place.

We would also like to thank all those involved in planning, funding and supporting the art therapy workshop at the University of Durban–Westville, KwaZulu–Natal, South Africa, and in particular, the participants for their keen interest, commitment and persistence in face of the changing South Africa and in light of their intense work schedules. Many thanks to Tessa Dally for supervision which proved integral to the creating of this workshop.

Thanks also to the following people for their help, support, input and expertise either in directly developing the project, or in helping us to advance our knowledge and experience:

- War Child, British non-government organisation working in Bosnia;
- Bosnian Support Group, British group directly supporting Hrastnik Camp;
- Misco Mimico, UNHCR Head of Social Services in Split, Croatia;
- Liz Palmer, the Art Works Trust, Durban, South Africa;
- Julie Manegold, Fine Art Department, University of Durban–Westville, South Africa;
- University of Durban–Westville, South Africa.

This is continuing work which is dependent on funds. We would like to also thank all those who show continued interest and desire to contribute in the future.

We are also grateful to HarperCollins Publishers for permission to reproduce the geographical statistics for the four countries mentioned in this report.

Summary

With continuing political crises in different parts of the globe, there is a growing awareness of the need to address the psychological effects of political conflict. The burden on the majority of local trained specialists who work with mental health has meant that in most cases there is a loss of, or depleted inherent support structure to deal with this.

There is now a greater recognition amongst those working in the context of political conflict that these problems exist and have enduring repercussions both for individuals involved and society at large (UNICEF, 1996; Smythe and Lewer, 1992; Sogoric, 1992; Medact, 1994; Gal, 1995; Modric, 1994; Garcia del Soto, 1994). Two surveys taken in 1994 demonstrate the enormity of the problem. A survey produced by the Department of Psychology, University of Natal, Pietermaritzburg, South Africa found that 84 per cent of black children in urban areas suffered from symptoms of post-traumatic stress disorder (PTSD) or major depression (Killian, 1994). A UNICEF survey of children in Sarajevo found that 23 per cent of children felt that life is not worth living (UNICEF, 1994).

In 1993, the number of people world-wide forced to leave their countries for fear of persecution and violence had risen to a total of 18.2 million. An average of nearly ten thousand people a day became refugees. In the former Yugoslavia alone nearly 4 million people have come to depend on international emergency assistance since late 1991 (UNHCR, 1993). The physical wounds of war are all too obvious, but as UNICEF quotes, the psychological wounds affect as many as 10 million children (1996, p. 1), many of whom grow up to perpetuate the violence they have experienced.

The situations that produce refugees also produce other forms of displacement and problems, including people who have not crossed an international border but face the same fears and resulting psychological difficulties as refugees.*

The term Post-traumatic Stress Disorder (PTSD)† is now a loosely and frequently used term in relation to the psychological consequences of political conflict. It is as a result of this that it is of vital importance that the centrality of the individual is remembered so that the response of mental health workers to trauma reactions does not become an institutional one. In the townships of KwaZulu–Natal, for example, although many children are displaying symptoms recognized as PTSD, it would be uncomfortable and perhaps even irresponsible to label all these children with the disorder, as it is a fallacy to assume that if something is wrong with society each individual is pathological.

However, although each individual who lives through war and political conflict will react differently, perhaps to the same chain of events, the experiences for all are real and most often overwhelming. In addition, studies of trauma do offer essential

*See 'The context: the former Yugoslavia. A psychological context', p. 22
†See Glossary

insight into the experience of the individual. 'There are many definitions of trauma, all have to do with being overwhelmed. At one level this is the experience of being overwhelmed by helpless, hopeless feelings, together with a whole mixture of undifferentiated emotions. The personality is temporarily put under immense stress and breaks down' (Melzak, 1992, p. 211).

In acknowledgement of the former, the Art Therapy Initiative (ATI) was established in 1994 in order to research and implement the setting up of an art therapy service for children, adults and caring professionals in the specific context of the former Yugoslavia – see Part II. The art therapy training workshops in South Africa grew out of and were informed by ATI's work and research in the former Yugoslavia.

Much has been learnt in recent years about the benefits that therapeutic work has to offer people who have lived through situations of political conflict, have been tortured, imprisoned or displaced. Nothing, of course, can compensate for the enormity of loss and trauma that many have experienced. Reflective work is no substitute for practical help such as primary healthcare, homes, welfare benefits, educational and occupational rehabilitation. However, the value of psychosocial methods of support is now widely accepted; amongst the services offered are: psychotherapy, counselling, psychology, occupational therapy, work therapy (UNICEF, 1996; Oxfam, 1996; Smythe and Lewer, 1992; Medact, 1994; Gal, 1995; Modric, 1994; Garcia del Soto, 1994).

In addition, the use of 'art as therapy' is recognised as of significant value *in the context of political conflict* (UNICEF, 1996; Oxfam, 1996; Smythe and Lewer, 1992; Medact, 1994; Sanderson, 1991; Golub, 1984; Seligman, 1991; Gregorian *et al.*, 1996; Klingman, Koenigsfeld and Markman, 1987). The purpose of art therapy is that it can provide a means of expression in the context of an experience which perhaps cannot yet be verbalised and is potentially overwhelming. In addition, the very nature of art draws on creativity and therefore dynamic, healthy elements of the individual.

Some of the benefits of art therapy include:

- Art-making is a shared language that crosses other language barriers.
- Art therapy demands active participation of the individual, combating apathy, boredom and alienation from refugee life, for example.
- The art-therapy process allows for catharsis – providing an appropriate and contained space in which to express any emotion.
- The concreteness of the art product may safely contain fears too 'dangerous' to say aloud.
- Art therapy fosters creativity – perhaps this could lead to 'living creatively' and being able to respond differently to a difficult situation.
- The art-making process is accessible to all ages.
- Art therapy is suitable for group work as well as individual.
- Art therapy can offer an alternative means of expression and communication.
- Art therapy is suitable for those who do not have mastery over verbal language.
- Art therapy can aid in increasing ability to concentrate.
- Art therapy can encourage choice and decision-making.
- Art therapy can increase self-respect and self-esteem.
- Art therapy is insight-oriented – leading to increased self-awareness, self-exploration and self-understanding, eventually leading to change.

- Involvement with art therapy enables the individual to cultivate influences supporting growth.

Art therapy combines both art and therapy. It is not possible or useful to separate art therapy into its individual components and therefore the benefits above overlap with other therapies while at the same time offering a unique therapeutic service.

What is art therapy?

Art therapy is a form of psychotherapy. In an art therapy session the individual is invited to draw, paint, sculpt. The focus in art therapy is on the image and the image-making in the presence of the therapist. At its centre is the understanding that this process can lead to change. Art therapy does not rely on previous or existing art skills.

The image in art therapy

The image or pictures in the session are seen as forms of, for example, imaginations, dreams, cognitions, thoughts, beliefs, memories and feelings. The images hold many meanings and may generate multiple interpretations. These can be reflected upon in depth and emphasis is placed on the meaning the individual gives to his/her image. *The image is not judged for technical or aesthetic competence.*

Who uses art therapy?

Art therapy is used in the National Health Service, community and private settings, social services, clinics, hospitals, prisons and schools with a wide range of clients. It may be offered on an individual or group basis to adults, young people or children depending on the needs of the client group and setting.

The art therapist

The art therapist is a trained professional, either with a postgraduate training or master's degree in art therapy and an initial degree in art or another relevant subject such as psychology. Individuals must have obtained relevant work experience in the caring professions before entry into an art therapy training and must show a continuing commitment to their personal art process.

Art-related projects are known to exist in situations of political conflict (UNICEF, 1996; Medact, 1994; Modric, 1994; Scottish European Aid, 1994; Marie Stopes International, 1996) in Croatia, Serbia, Bosnia, Angola, Rwanda, Romania and the Philippines. These range from writing and poetry projects to music, drama, performance art and mural painting. However, these art projects should not be confused with the continuing therapeutic support created through the discipline of art therapy (Sanderson, 1995; Golub, 1984; Seligman, 1995; Skripchenko, 1996; Klingman, Koenigsfeld and Markman, 1987). Although documentation exists on projects carried out by individual art therapists there has, to date, been no collation of this material.

This book attempts in part to address this shortcoming through pilot art therapy projects, research and bibliographies. It also outlines useful practical information as well as accounts of obstacles and ways to take the work further, without which individuals and organisations may continue to repeat isolated pieces of research and to make, rather than redress, mistakes.

Based upon on-site field work, research, interviews and literature reviews, the Art Therapy Initiative presents this book in three parts, Parts II and III forming the basis for Part I:

Part I: the presentation of *two models* developed in response to identified need in the former Yugoslavia and South Africa respectively and which provide a base for art therapy work in comparable situations.

Model 1: for the development of an art therapy service for children and adults in the context of political conflict or war.
Model 2: for art therapy workshops for local professionals and carers already working with people who have directly experienced violence.

Part II: *detailed research* on pilot art therapy projects and fieldwork in the former Yugoslavia (Bosnia, Croatia, Slovenia).

Part III: *a report* on the Art Therapy Initiative's art therapy workshops held at the University of Durban–Westville, KwaZulu–Natal (South Africa).

All three parts form a complete book and should be read as such, in conjunction with the references and bibliographies.

The provision of an art therapy service in the context of political conflict enables different sections of the community to benefit from a creative process, within which each individual's concerns can be acknowledged. The hope is that, through the artwork and the witnessed story, the internal experience of the external situation can be attended to now, in this generation, so as not to carry it on to the next.

The Art Therapy Initiative

Introduction

The Art Therapy Initiative (ATI) is an independent London-based art and art therapy service established in 1994 by Debra Kalmanowitz and Bobby Lloyd, registered art therapists. To date, ATI has been supported by private sponsors, the Bosnian Support Group, War Child, the Art Psychotherapy Unit, Goldsmiths' College, London University and the University of Durban–Westville and the Art Works Trust, KwaZulu–Natal, South Africa.

The primary aims of the Art Therapy Initiative are:
1. To offer an art and art therapy service in the context of political conflict to children, adults and caring professionals.
2. To offer individual and group art therapy in London to children, adults and families who have fled political conflict.
3. To offer training and support to carers and professionals working in the context of political conflict.
4. To undertake research into the above where and when it would directly contribute to the work and enhance the understanding of the subject for art therapists and related professionals.
5. To communicate understanding and insights gained and enter into a discourse with a wider audience through workshops, exhibitions, seminars and delivery of papers at conferences.

The origins of the initiative

This work in the former Yugoslavia began in November 1993 with an idea conceived by War Child, a British charity whose work focused on Bosnia. War Child had identified the scope of personal suffering as a result of its work in Bosnia and identified art therapy as potentially having an important contribution to make in this regard. War Child therefore decided to investigate establishing what they called an 'arts-based trauma centre', which would offer the arts therapies as central to their programme. In November 1993, War Child contacted Dr Diane Waller, head of the Art Psychotherapy Unit at Goldsmiths' College, London University, seeking professional advice. Advertisements seeking interested art therapists were also placed in the *Artists Newsletter* and *The Newsletter* of the British Association of Art Therapists. In February 1994, fortnightly meetings, based at Goldsmiths' College, were subsequently set up to begin exploring the viability and implementation of such a project and recruit art therapists to carry out the work.

In the initial exploratory stages, War Child regularly shifted the location for the 'arts-based trauma centre' between Sarajevo, the Dalmatian Coast and East Mostar. To date, the project has changed its focus and War Child is in the process of funding and supervising the building of the Pavarotti Music Centre in Mostar, having secured substantial funds for this particular project. This will hold performance and arts-based therapy rooms, a recording studio and community space. In addition, they are funding an orphanage in Tusla and have begun to work internationally.

In late 1994, ATI was established with a small working party with Dr Diane Waller as consultant, and a representative from War Child amongst its members. ATI carried out two pilot art therapy projects in Slovenia and Croatia, and research in London, Croatia and Bosnia (Sarajevo and East Mostar) – following up connections already established by War Child and the Art Psychotherapy Unit in Croatia and Bosnia, in addition to making new ones. By 1995, War Child had committed itself to the Music School and ATI continued its work independently from War Child while remaining associated with the Art Psychotherapy Unit, receiving a Research Grant from Goldsmiths' College, London University to consolidate research and collate findings.

Overview of the work of the initiative

The Art Therapy Initiative, former Yugoslavia, 1994–96

The Art Therapy Initiative worked on this project based in the former Yugoslavia from 1994 to 1996. This timescale enabled ATI to accommodate the erratic situation of war in the former Yugoslavia, the sporadic acquisition of funds for the work (much of the work has been carried out without funding) and to allow for time to gather and collate material. On-site work in the former Yugoslavia itself took place over three visits in 1994. This included two pilot art therapy projects – the first in Slovenia over five weeks and reaching 200 Bosnian and Croatian refugees (of whom 100 were children), the second in Croatia over three weeks and reaching 24 Bosnian refugees (of whom 21 were children and 3 were mothers).

Formal interviews with organisations and individual professionals in the former Yugoslavia involved 20 meetings in Zagreb and Split, Croatia, and East Mostar and Sarajevo, Bosnia.

The above work was funded by private sponsorship, the Bosnian Support Group, War Child and Goldsmiths' College, London University.

The Art Therapy Initiative, Kwazulu–Natal, South Africa, 1995

The Art Therapy Initiative worked on a time-based project in KwaZulu–Natal, South Africa over a period of five months from September 1995 to January 1996. ATI was invited to South Africa by the Art Works Trust. This is a small South African-based non-profit, non-government organisation working primarily with young people in KwaZulu–Natal who have grown up in a climate of violence. The Art Works Trust 'encourages self-expression and creativity' and offers a variety of art projects in the townships.

The Art Works Trust saw the work of, and experience gained by ATI in the former Yugoslavia as relevant to the situation in KwaZulu–Natal, despite the clear differences.

ATI devised and facilitated a four-week experiential art therapy workshop for professionals working with children and adults in KwaZulu–Natal, who have directly experienced violence. The course took place from 22 November to 16 December, 1995 and involved 9 core participants. The workshops included experiential groups, case consultations and site visits to places of work. Integral were supervision groups that focused on participants' work, discussing ways in which insights gained could be implemented into this. In addition, a further 15 interested professionals and carers attended seminars open to a wider audience and offered for the duration of the course. Implicit was the understanding that ATI educate a wider audience on the benefits of art therapy particularly in the context of political conflict. This took the form of six interviews to newspapers and radio and an exhibition at an art centre in Durban on art and art therapy in the former Yugoslavia.

Also integral and important to the course was a commitment by the participants to pass on insights gained to colleagues and others working in the field. The project outcomes are being monitored by the University of Durban–Westville as part of the community outreach programme initiated by Dr N D Zuma, Minister of Health, South Africa.

The above work was funded by the Art Works Trust and the University of Durban–Westville, KwaZulu–Natal, South Africa, with flights donated by British Airways.

The Art Therapy Initiative, London, 1995–96

London-based interviews

This aspect of the work involved interviews with London-based organisations including:

- the Medical Foundation for the Care of Victims of Torture.
- B-H Woman (a Croatian women's organisation).
- The Serious Road Trip (British non-government organisation – in the former Yugoslavia).
- UK JAID (United Kingdom Jewish Aid and International Development).
- ODA (Overseas Development Administration).
- Humanarty (London-based organisation – collating art-related work in humanitarian aid, now called Creative Rights Forum).
- Professionals working with refugees at the Tavistock Clinic.
- the Bosnian Advisory Centre (centre for Bosnian refugees in West London).
- War Child.
- Goldsmiths' College – the Art Psychotherapy Unit.
- Consultations with the working party, Dr Diane Waller and senior art therapists.
- The Bosnian Support Group.
- RAW (Returning Aid Workers).
- Continuing dialogue with organisations and research into existing art and art therapy projects in the former Yugoslavia as they have developed and information has become available.*

Literature review

A review of related literature has served to enhance ATI's understanding of the work overall.†

ATI workshops, lectures and exhibitions

ATI has facilitated experiential workshops, lectured on art therapy courses, delivered papers on its work and mounted exhibitions.

*See Part II: 'Update 1996'.
†See Part II: 'Literature review'.

PART I: PROJECT PROPOSALS

Model 1: An art therapy service for children and adults
as developed for the former Yugoslavia

This model is based on art therapy work and related research carried out in the context of the former Yugoslavia.
This model can provide a structure for establishing small art therapy services in the context of political conflict or war. See also p. 73.

The target group

The target group is children and adults: refugees, locally displaced people and people who have directly experienced violence.

The aims

The project aims to offer art therapy in areas of need. Although 'art sessions' can provide support while war is continuing, for 'art therapy' per se, a degree of stability needs to be in place as a minimum requirement. A reliable structure and clarification from the outset of the parameters within which the work is to take place is essential.*

Immediate aims would include the provision of:
- Art therapy for groups and individuals: short and long term.
- Training and guidelines, consultation for local workers who use or could make use of art in their work.
- Psychological support for local workers. Support is essential as it is acknowledged that burn-out is widespread and energies need to be replenished.†
- Handing over the art therapy service to local bodies as soon as possible.

The 5–10-year aims

This would involve extension into a 5–10-year project, depending on local circumstances and financial support. Therapeutic work demands reliability and continuity. A long-term project would enable a therapeutic process to be of great benefit to individuals and could include:
- Setting in place a structure in which art therapists from outside the country can work alongside and contribute to the needs of local professionals.
- The development of a local art therapy training programme. This could be facilitated by a related professional body.
- The translation of art therapy literature into the local language.
- An extension of the service to involve other expressive arts therapies – drama, music, dance.

*In the circumstances of the former Yugoslavia, for example, art therapy can now take place as the former Yugoslavia is in a 'post-war' phase in which re-development has begun.
†See Model 2.

- Continuing and long-term research in the field which could inform and be further applied to other areas.

Staffing structure
Project co-ordinators

There should be two project co-ordinators who will be responsible for overseeing the art therapy service(s). They will work half-time (the equivalent of two-and-a-half days each week, including block visits to project locations). This will enable sharing of roles and responsibilities.

The following forms the outline of a job description:
Each chosen project co-ordinator must:
- have an ability to work on their own initiative as well as part of a team
- have the ability to prioritise their own workload
- be able to respond creatively to difficult situations
- be willing to work through interpreters where necessary
- have clear project management experience
- have experience of setting up community-based programmes
- have proven organisational ability
- have excellent communication skills.

The following would be desirable:
- be trained as an art therapist with a recognised art therapy training body
- have reached Senior One Level
- have had at least three years' working experience in the field of art therapy
- be computer-literate.

The co-ordinator's role should include an on-site planning period for:
(i) Identifying and establishing appropriate local work locations.

(ii) Finding living accommodation for art therapists, where needed.

(iii) Liaising with local professionals on site (teachers, social workers, nurses, interpreters).

(iv) Setting up the minimum requirements for an art therapy service:
- Identifying and establishing appropriate minimum requirements: regular room/working space; access to water; work surfaces; seating; light.
- Locating local art suppliers.
- Developing administrative structures. Implementing these locally – filing systems, access to fax and/telephone, etc.
- Negotiating appropriate time period for art therapy work.
- Identifying local supervision and support networks.
- Setting up the initial stages of a referral system.
- Formalising documentation.

'Home'-based work should include:
(i) Monitoring and evaluation of the project overall – including regular communication with each art therapy team, assessment of regular reports (minimum, three-monthly) and regular meetings with the advisory committee.

(ii) Responsibility for centralising all resources, including literature, reports received, etc.

(iii) Home-based orientation workshops for therapists going out to the location.

(iv) Recruitment of art therapists, with the Advisory Committee and specialist consultants.

Art therapists

Minimum of two art therapists, working as a team. It is important that art therapists work in pairs.

- Art therapy groups can be larger, therefore more people reached.
- One therapist can provide consistency in case of sickness or absence.
- Psychological work can often be very intensive. It is accepted practice in the discipline of art therapy for art therapists to work together in order to provide support and peer supervision. In a situation in which formal support and supervision are unavailable, this is essential.

The following forms the outline of a job description:

(i) Each chosen art therapist must:
- be trained as an art therapist with a recognised art therapy training body
- have reached Senior One Level
- have had at least three years' working experience in the field of art therapy
- have an ability to work on their own initiative as well as part of a team
- be able to respond creatively to difficult situations
- be willing to work with interpreters where necessary. In this case, clear structures need to be clarified and confidentiality adhered to.

(ii) The minimum time commitment should be three months and the maximum time should be one year.

(iii) The art therapists should work within a team of two, and together devise and deliver the specific programme to meet the needs of the local situation. This will be in dialogue with the project co-ordinators, local management and local support services and based on the art therapy structure provided:
- The art therapists must suit their programme to the time-frame for which they are committed. (i.e. three or six months/one year)
- The art therapists need to take a period of time to observe, meet with workers and evaluate needs of the individuals in the particular situation, for example, which individuals are suited to group therapy and which individuals would only benefit from individual sessions etc.
- The therapists would be expected to work five days a week. The days would be typically divided into art therapy sessions, progress report writing, attendance at meetings.

(iv) The art therapists should undertake the following:
- Group and individual art therapy sessions with children and adults.
- Consultations for local professionals and carers.
- Assessments, referrals, responsibility for case-loads. These would involve follow-up meetings with family/carer/institution, where applicable.

(v) The art therapists should work, where possible, as members of the local multi-disciplinary team and participate in regular/weekly meetings, where possible.

(vi) The art therapist should be required to monitor and evaluate their work through the keeping of process notes, regular clinical reports, and photographic documentation.

(vi) Where there is no local supervision structure, a regular time must be built into the programme for peer supervision.

(viii) The art therapists must be responsible for an art materials budget, and the maintenance of appropriate supplies, through local suppliers, where possible.

Art therapy consultants

(i) Art therapy consultants should form part of the committee for selection of art therapists.

(ii) A specialist consultant to the project would offer overall support and consultancy to the project co-ordinators.

(iii) Follow-up supervision to art therapists returning from their work should be offered by art therapists.

(iv) The consultants (and other practitioners) should also be invited to run short block-workshops on location for local carers and professionals, where appropriate.

Advisory committee

The advisory committee should meet at regular intervals to evaluate the overall work of the project and discuss general policy. The members should include members of the original working party, other interested practitioners and related professionals.

Local staffing

Use of local interpreters will be necessary in the following:
- Meetings with local professionals who do not speak English.
- One-to-one art therapy sessions in which the individual does not speak English.
- Group art therapy sessions in which there is no English-speaking participant.
- Consultation and support sessions in which there is no English-speaking participant.

Experience shows that at most times there is someone available and willing to speak English. At times when this is not appropriate, an interpreter will also be necessary.

All local art therapy work should take place in communication with/alongside local carers and professionals.

The art therapy structure

(i) Minimum time-frame for art therapists to work is three months. This is a satisfactory period of time for 'brief' therapy work. The time-frame established at the outset should be adhered to.

(ii) The art therapy service should be offered five days each week.

(iii) Continuity
Structures need to be set in place to enable each time block (three months/six months, etc.)
to be followed by a further time block (if applicable, art therapists to work in rotation).

(iv) The maximum period for art therapy work is one year. This is to prevent burn-out.

(v) A typical week should include:
- group art therapy
- individual art therapy
- supervision by local professionals or peer supervision (once a week).
- meeting with local workers involved with those receiving art therapy (once a week).
- psychological support/consultation for local professionals and carers
- participation at other meetings which are part of the existing structure.
- report-writing, documentation.
- meetings with family/carer/institution, where appropriate.

(vi) Confidentiality
Confidentiality is integral to all art therapy work.

(vii) Group art therapy
Art therapy groups are used in a variety of settings (community, hospital, prison,
school) and seen as an effective form of therapy. An advantage of group therapy is
that group members may support each other and learn from their peers. This could
be useful in the context of refugee centres, for example, where individuals who are
separated from their families and homes may feel isolated and alone. The fact that
group therapy can reach greater numbers of individuals at one time is of particular
importance in the context of war in which therapeutic support services are in most
cases stretched to their limits.

There are two types of group relevant to this context:
- The *open group* is run each week at the same time for any individual who chooses to
  join or is referred. In this group the membership is constantly changing and the
  therapeutic benefits of the group such as sharing and trust are sometimes not
  possible. In the context of populations that are transient or unstable, this group
  structure can be useful and can serve to provide valuable therapeutic support.
- The *closed group* is run each week at the same time for individuals who are referred.
  The group is closed to others and therefore the membership remains constant. In
  this group, a 'group culture' can develop and trust can be established. The
  individual will therefore gain from both the art process and the group process and
  the therapeutic work has potential to be developed in a greater depth. In this
  context, this group structure is particularly beneficial in situations where the
  population is relatively stable.

(viii) Individual art therapy
One-to-one art therapy offers individuals who are unable to be part of a group a
confidential, regular and reliable space in which to begin to look at their problems.
For some, their experiences, for example, may make it impossible to start to work on
personal concerns in a group for fear of being exposed, or the information being used

against them. Individual art therapy may also be useful for those with complex problems which might include difficulties in functioning in groups.

There is a place for both individual art therapy and group art therapy and this would address the different needs of the individuals using the art therapy service as well as of the local context. The majority of the work will take place in groups although individual therapy sessions should be available where necessary and possible.

(ix) Consultation
Consultation can be offered to local professionals already using art in their work or planning to use art in their role as carers.

In addition a support group may be offered, where appropriate.

Monitoring and evaluation

(i)   The art therapists should be required to monitor and evaluate their work through the keeping of standardised forms, process notes, regular clinical reports and photographic documentation.

(ii) The co-ordinators should be responsible for the monitoring and evaluation of the project overall – including regular communication with each art therapy team, assessment of each (three monthly) report and regular meetings with the advisory committee.

(iii) Supervision (including peer supervision) will be an integral part of the work.

(iv) An annual report should be required from each art therapy team, where applicable, and from the project co-ordinators.

Organisational structure – implementation options

(i)   An independent art therapy project – funded by an aid/other organisation.

(ii) Art therapists to be employed by an aid organisation as part of its staffing structure, based on the model provided.

(iii) Art therapists to work as freelance workers.

Financial forecast

The full budget to be prepared in advance should take into account the following areas based on the duration of the project:

(i)   Art therapists: salaries and expenses.

(ii) Project co-ordinators: salaries and expenses.

(iii) Consultancy fees: for home-based supervision and consultation.

(iv) Administration: local and home-based costs. These include: telephone/fax; stationery; printing.

(v) Documentation: clinical work – slides/photographs; research and development of an archive (articles; literature).

(vi) Materials: basic materials to be bought locally as far as possible, within an allocated budget.

(vii) Interpreters: based on local figures, as the need arises.

(viii) Contingency: to allow for unforeseen costs.

Model 2: Art therapy workshops for local professionals and carers
as developed for KwaZulu–Natal, South Africa

This model was developed for professionals who work with people who have
directly experienced violence in KwaZulu–Natal, South Africa.
The model provides the structure for training local professionals and carers in the use of art in their work. See also p. 73.

This model offers not only workshops in the use of art but also the chance for
participants to replenish depleted energies. This four-week workshop intends to
provide participants with insights into the use of art in their work – drawing on each
individual's intrinsic professional and academic knowledge and skills. The
participants are committed, where possible, to carry these insights into their work as
well as to pass them on to others working in the field.
This model is not a 'training' and therefore does not provide a qualification to practise as art therapists.

The target group

This model is aimed at professionals and carers working in the context of political
conflict* and can be adapted for people with some experience of mental health issues
but no formal training.

The aims of the workshop

(i)   To provide an intensive experience of art and art-making for individual
       participants as part of a group which will hopefully lead to insights that will
       resonate in their work.

(ii)   To provide a forum which will bring a wide concept of art and art therapy as a
       basis for continuing questioning with which participants can continue to work.

Both (i) and (ii) are intended to contribute to:
- building confidence in using art materials and in the image-making process;
- a richer understanding of the potential of the different art media;
- a greater understanding of group-work and therapeutic group process;

*All the participants in the KwaZulu–Natal workshop had some formal training in mental health issues and
were working in the field. This was important for enabling the workshops to have a longer ongoing life: as a
result of their background training, integration of the art therapy insights into their existing knowledge was
possible as was the passing of insights learnt to other workers in the field. The professionals came from such
diverse backgrounds as nursing, psychology, counselling, teaching and the arts. This range contributed to the
richness of the workshop and the sharing of professional knowledge, which was seen as integral.

- sensitivity to 'emotional indicators'; the limitations of interpretation of art-work;
- some understanding of principles, theory and application of art therapy.

(iii) To provide a forum in which the wealth of knowledge, skills and experience of participants can be shared. Sharing of professional knowledge is integral.

(iv) To provide an opportunity for personal learning and for replenishing depleted energies.

(v) To define with the participants insights and skills learnt throughout the course. (These will be passed on to other workers and can be assimilated into their own work.)

The staffing structure

Art therapist facilitators

There should be two art therapist facilitators because:
- co-work is an effective way of working in groups and imparting this workshop model of training.
- groups can be larger.
- peer supervision is essential for this work.

Local administrative staff

An administrative support system for the workshop needs to be set up as far as possible prior to the arrival of the facilitators. Solid groundwork facilitates smooth running of the workshop. The minimum requirement involves centralised responsibility on site by a staff member familiar with the administrative system, secretarial and general technical support. The allocation of clear responsibility with identified channels of communication is necessary for the smooth day-to-day running of the workshop.

The following local staff support would be desirable:
- secretarial support for general administration;
- an assistant for photocopying and general duties;
- a technician for provision and maintenance of materials and equipment.

Art therapy consultant

The art therapist facilitators should attend a period of supervision from a senior art therapist prior to the workshops as well as on their return. This is essential for support and guidance in enabling the facilitators to devise and structure the workshop to suit the specific needs of the context, as well as to evaluate the outcomes.

The art therapy structure

The workshops are structured on an *'experiential' model* (that is, learning by experiencing through doing) which is understood to be an effective way to teach about the process of art therapy.

Art and the art-making process need to be allowed a time and a place. The importance of this is often overlooked, or dismissed as 'non-work' or 'non-productive'. This workshop model addresses this by providing each participant with the time and the space in which to engage and immerse themselves in art-making. It is hoped that each participant's personal experience will provide them with ideas, insights and skills which will resonate in their work.

- The participants should be committed to attend the workshop for the full day, four days each week, over a four-week period. The facilitators are committed to visiting areas in which participants work on two days each week in an attempt to gain greater understanding of the specifics of the local situation.

- All experiential work to be supported by theoretical seminars as well as written material which will be included in a package handed out at the beginning of the workshop.* *A combination of experiential workshops with theoretical discussions and literature is effective and serves as an identified method of teaching art therapy.*

Workshop schedule

Times	Wednesday	Thursday	Friday	Saturday
8.30–9.30	Interactive art therapy group	Interactive art therapy group	Interactive art therapy group	Interactive art therapy group
9.30–10.00	Coffee	Coffee	Coffee	Coffee
10.00–12.00	Open studio	Materials workshop*	Case conference	Open studio
12.00–1.30	Lunch	Lunch	Lunch	Lunch
1.30–3.30	Open studio	Articles discussion	Theme workshop	Seminar
3.30–4.00	Plenary	Plenary	Plenary	Plenary

Art therapy groups can take many different forms. The style of group depends on a number of elements – the style and the theoretical persuasion of the art therapist, the place or circumstance of work, the timescale available in which to work and the goal towards which the art therapy is working, to name a few. Because the participants of the art therapy workshops are as varied as the clients with whom they work and circumstances in which they work, it is useful to include different experiences of art therapy. As is clear from the above schedule, four different styles of art therapy workshops could be included; an *Open art therapy Studio*, an *Interactive art therapy Group*, a *Materials Workshop* and a *Theme Workshop* together with articles, seminars and case consultations.†

Setting and space

The space provided must be appropriate for the workshop's needs. It should ideally have the following: adequate light, running water, storage space, wall space, tables, chairs, easels, washable floors and toilet facilities.

*In the South Africa workshop, a different material (clay, drawing, painting, scrap) was explored each week. Articles related to these materials were included in the package provided.
†For workshop definitions see Part III, p. 79.

Materials and equipment

The materials are to be provided locally, where possible.* The categories included: paint; dry materials; paper; glues and fixative; brushes; clay; scrap.

Size of the group

Fourteen is the maximum size for the group in relation to this experiential method of learning.†

Visits

An important part of the facilitators' role is to visit participants' places of work. This is fundamental in understanding of context.

Guest lecturers

Use of local professionals as guest lecturers or workshop facilitators in the art therapy workshops would enable a network of local knowledge to be shared and developed within the context of art therapy.

Monitoring methods for evaluation

(i) Documentation
All art-work to be documented through slides and/or photographic film.

(ii) Process notes
All workshops and groups to be recorded by the facilitators through process notes.

(iii) Questionnaires
Confidential questionnaires to be handed out and filled in on the first day of the course.

(iv) Evaluations
Confidential evaluations to be handed out and filled in on the last day of the course.

(v) Long-term evaluations
Due to the style of the workshop an interval of a six- to twelve-month period is useful before sending out longer-term evaluations.** Participants will be asked to comment on if/how/where they are using insights and skills gained during the course, and for comments/suggestions at this stage.

(vi) Supervision
This could take two forms:
- 'Home'-based, for a period prior to the workshops with a senior art therapist. This could be used by the facilitators in devising and structuring the course, and on their return in evaluating it.

*In South Africa, the collection of scrap materials by participants was an integral element of the workshop.
†In South Africa, as a result of practical limitations, there were nine participants.
**In KwaZulu–Natal, long-term evaluations were required from participants by the University of Durban–Westville one year after the workshops took place.

- Peer supervision throughout the course, between the facilitators, to monitor the progress of the workshops, and offer support and guidance.

Follow-up

This model represents a focused, short-term training workshop and can therefore stand on its own. However, follow-up to the workshops is seen as important.*

The following are options for follow-up:

(i) Pair-work
Participants to divide into pairs and to work together to introduce art into their different work situations. The pair-work is suggested for support, sharing of knowledge and peer supervision.

(ii) Regular group meetings
These are suggested to offer support and to carry on the momentum. Dates can be fixed during the final days of the workshop.

(iii) Collaboration with local artists
In order to implement insights/skills: the artists and group members working together to offer art therapeutically.

(iv) 'Expanding Circles'
These could be based on a scheme successfully used in follow-up to a training seminar in Israel offered to stress-workers from the former Yugoslavia. The 'Expanding Circles' would involve subsequent follow-up in-country training workshops instructed by the participants, *and closely supervised by the facilitators (or prepared with their help)*. The workshops would take the form of small seminars in which the material learned could be shared with a broader circle of local workers (Gal 1995).

(v) Follow-up visits
These could be offered by art therapists and take the following forms:
- Supervision of those who have already participated in art therapy workshops.
- Further art therapy workshops for the same and/or new participants. These could be run by art therapists from outside or within the locality/country in which the workshops take place.

Financial forecast

The full budget needs to be prepared in advance to take into account the following areas based on the duration of the project:

(i) Salaries of art therapist facilitators, to cover: workshop fees; preparation; final report; follow-up.

*In relation to the *Helping the Helpers Project* (Gal, 1995), it was found that the greatest downfall of the training was that the individuals trained became stuck with what they had learnt and did not know how to take this further. They began to practise skills learnt by rote which lost their value. Supervision and follow-up bridged this until the next training was possible.

(ii) Expenses of art therapist facilitators, to cover local costs: accommodation; internal travel; return air flight; living expenses.

(iii) Consultancy fees, for supervision and consultancy: provided by a senior art therapist for a period before and after the workshop.

(iv) Basic materials: to be bought locally as far as possible, within an allocated budget.

(v) Administration: local and home-based costs. These include: telephone /fax; stationery; printing; postage.

(vi) Costs to cover slide and photographic film, processing and printing, video, etc. to document the workshops where appropriate.

(vii) Interpreters: based on local figures, as the need arises.

(viii) Contingency: to allow for unforeseen costs, such as hiring of equipment.

PART II: RESEARCH DOCUMENT: ART THERAPY IN THE FORMER YUGOSLAVIA

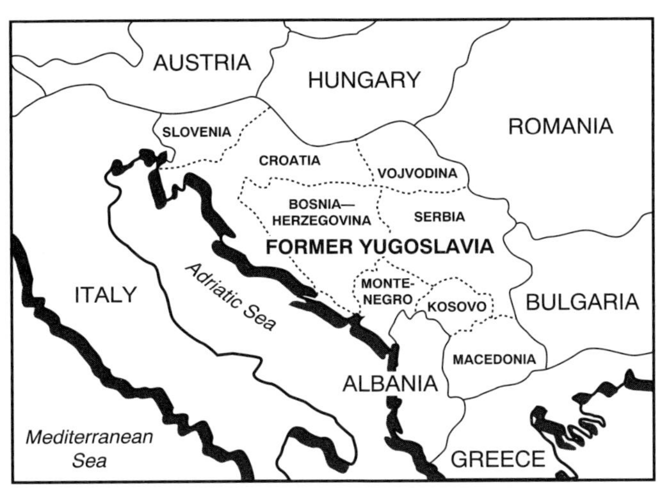

Abstract

This document is based upon projects and research carried out between January 1994 and June 1996. It attempts to identify the role for individuals that art and art therapy has to play in responding to the psychological impact of the war in Bosnia, Croatia and Slovenia.

Data were gathered from interviews, observation, on-site pilot art therapy projects and field work.

Conclusions of this research carried out by the Art Therapy Initiative (ATI) demonstrate that there is immense scope and use for art therapy in the 'post-war phase'.

Methodology

This is a qualitative study which would be defined primarily as 'action research'. The study is concerned with understanding the perspective of the individual, to seek insight rather than statistical analysis and the approach is essentially a practical, problem-solving one. ATI formulated tentative, general principles in relation to the problems already identified by War Child; from these principles, hypotheses were generated about what action was likely to lead to the establishment and collection of information required. Such actions as interviews, observation, on-site pilot art therapy projects, and field-work were carried out. This included sharing of the same experience as the individuals so as to understand better, as far as was possible, their situation and added some elements of the 'ethnographic style' of research which was an integral and important part of the therapeutic understanding.

The on-site pilot art therapy projects took place in two contrasting refugee centres in Slovenia and Croatia. This work consisted of what ATI called 'art sessions' and introduced art therapy. The length of the projects was short and therefore limited but valuable in assessing the responses and potential for art therapy in this context.

In *Slovenia,* the refugee centre is located in Hrastnik, a mining town. The population in the centre has remained consistent – more or less – for four years. This consists of two hundred people of whom one hundred were children. Art sessions in different forms were offered to all groups in the centre over two periods.

In *Croatia,* the refugee centre is located on an island off the Dalmatian Coast called Prvic. The centre is a place of transition with the population constantly shifting. At the time of the pilot project, the centre consisted of 24 people of whom 21 were children and 3 were mothers. Art sessions in different forms were offered to all age groups in the centre over a three-week period.

This research document is a collection and assessment of the material gathered and used to revise the earlier hypotheses and to modify and formulate the development of the proposal for establishing an art therapy service in the former Yugoslavia.

An important feature of this work as an action research is that the task is not finished despite the fact that this specific research is complete.

Aims and purposes of the study

This research document is a response to repeated requests from organisations, professionals and local people with whom ATI met during research visits in Slovenia, Bosnia and Croatia in 1994.

The feasibility of art therapy in the former Yugoslavia

The Art Therapy Initiative (ATI) aimed to research the feasibility of art therapy in the context of the former Yugoslavia and asked the following questions:
- Is there a place for art therapy in the context of this war?
- Is art therapy relevant to the context of the former Yugoslavia?
- What psycho-social services are already in existence?
- Could art therapy provide something that is not already being offered?
- Local feedback: is art therapy wanted and needed?
- Who would most benefit from it?
- Where should the project be located?
- What is the possibility of setting up a working structure?

Research into existing art and art therapy projects

ATI aimed to gather as much information as was possible on existing art and art therapy projects, both through interviews of local and international aid organisations in the former Yugoslavia, and subsequently in the UK. In 1994, aid was sporadic and there was no centralised information system. It was therefore difficult for research to be comprehensive. Subsequently in 1996, questionnaires were sent to aid organisations involved in the former Yugoslavia. Although a number responded through providing information on art and art therapy projects only one organisation returned the questionnaire (see 'Update 1996').

Art therapy pilot projects

ATI provided short-term 'art sessions', introducing art therapy into two different refugee centres, at Hrastnik in Slovenia and Prvic in Croatia. The overall aim was to bring art to the refugee centres and to assess if and how art therapy could be used in this context.

The context: the former Yugoslavia

A psychological context

After four-and-a-half years of war in the former Yugoslavia the psychological impact of the war is widespread and the support structure that once existed is now fragmented. The situation of war is an extreme one. Families and individuals have lost their homes, have witnessed death close by, have been in situations in which they thought they would be killed and feared for their lives. The cost of war on the entire population is clearly vast and far reaching.

Investigations have been carried out by a number of aid organizations on the subject of 'trauma reactions' to war and point to the complexity and multi-faceted nature of the subject. UNICEF for example, has attempted to understand the reactions to, and the psychological effects of war on children in the former Yugoslavia. In looking into this, UNICEF psychologists carried out a psychological survey of school-age children in Sarajevo, Bosnia in 1994* and found the following:

- 23 per cent of children had been forced to leave their own town or village during the war;
- 7 per cent of children reported that family members had been wounded or killed during the war;
- 46 per cent had seen dead bodies;
- 79 per cent had been in a situation during the war in which they thought they would be killed;
- 97 per cent had experienced shelling very near by;
- 96 per cent had had their homes attacked or shelled;
- 55 per cent had been shot at by snipers;
- 11 per cent had experienced serious food and water shortage.

Out of the same sample taken in Sarajevo, reactions showed that '23 per cent of children thought that life was not worth living; 29 per cent felt unbearable sorrow; 21 per cent felt alone; 20 per cent had terrifying dreams and 34 per cent had stomach aches; this may be evidence of extreme hunger, or may be psychosomatically conditioned'. UNICEF also noted that 'children's trauma reactions were not only linked to their direct war experiences: among children who had feared death from cold or hunger, these were the strongest factors explaining their psychological suffering' (UNICEF, *Annual Report*, 1994a, p. 12).

In many parts of the region care providers themselves have been severely affected and in addition to this there has been a drain of local caring professionals and

---

*Data were collated by sampling 1,505 primary school children in Sarajevo in June and July of 1993 (see Appendix 1 for survey of children in Mostar).

specialists from most of the big cities. As a result, many positions were filled by inexperienced individuals who themselves were traumatized, burnt-out and in need of training but who nevertheless demonstrated extraordinary commitment.

Although many individuals are overwhelmed by their experience only some will develop PTSD. The essential feature of this disorder defined by the DSM (*Diagnostic and Statistical Manual of Mental Disorders*) is the development of characteristic symptoms following a psychologically distressing event that is outside the range of common human experience. These symptoms involve re-experiencing the traumatic event, avoidance of stimuli associated with the event, numbing of general responsiveness and increased arousal.

Although ATI was and is aware of the scale of the problem, its intention and hope was to begin to address at least a small part of it through direct work with children, adults and carers involving art or therapy groups, training and research.

A theoretical context

Art therapy in the context of war

The concept of art as therapy in the context of war is not new. A handful of related articles explore the role of art therapy in a range of diverse but related situations. These include for example: art in concentration camps, art therapy with survivors of torture, with Vietnam combat veterans and art therapy in relation to trauma generally. Most of the articles discuss long-term art therapy work and talk about the role it plays in integrating the war experience into the lives of the individuals with whom the therapists work. That the individual is made to feel less than human as a result of their war experience, whether it be having to flee, having to fight or being tortured – as participants or recipients – and that through the art the individual can be helped to regain their humanity is an idea that runs through the literature.

Zivya Seligman (1991) writes about the spontaneous emergence of theatre activities which was not an isolated phenomenon in even the worst of the concentration camps. 'Africa Express' (a programme on British Channel Four television in April 1995) showed that in one Rwandan refugee camp in Zaire drumming has emerged as a group activity amongst the youth which has amongst other things served to positively redirect their energies. When ATI visited Sarajevo, they met art students who had daily risked crossing 'snipers' alley' in order to get to their studio at the art school on the other side of the river. ATI was invited by one mother to see the room of her daughter, also a student, who had covered all four walls with her diary of her experience of a year of the war – poems, words, posters and drawings. Seligman writes: 'I perceive the theatre activity that characterised most of the concentration camps as part of the [same] struggle for life. If we could explain what sustained the drive to live in a setting that offered little realistic hope for survival, we might be able to explain what sustained this extraordinary drive to create, to perform, or to be a spectator in this very same setting' (Seligman, 1991, p. 125).

In the context of arts therapies, art is used consciously to reach individuals and groups beyond the 'artists' in the community, in order to facilitate expression and aid individuals to eventually come to terms with and integrate their experience.

The role of *witness* is important in understanding art therapy work in this context. Malcolm Learmonth explores the concept and the function of 'witness' in art therapy. He writes: 'an unwitnessed story will tend to become stuck, and tell itself again'. Learmonth expands on the term as that which 'neither denies and represses the traumatic material, nor is possessed by it'. The image and the image-making enable the experience to be present and seen, 'to be authentic, without being overwhelming'. 'A precondition of witness is presence. Another may be suspending judgement. This is the art of conveying to the client that they are really being seen and heard in an active and interactive way' (Learmonth, 1994, pp. 19–21).

In this context of refugee camps and war where art sessions played a supportive therapeutic role, a witnessing and maintaining presence was often the only intervention possible.

Bosnia report

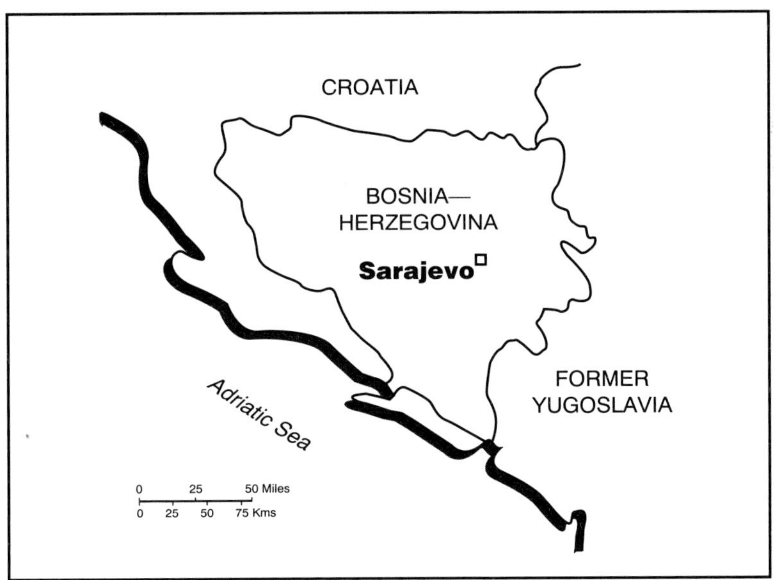

Figure 1: **Map of Bosnia, 1996**

The Republic of Bosnia–Herzegovina, 1996

Status   Republic
Area   51,131 sq km (9,736 sq miles)
Population   3,707,000
Capital   Sarajevo
Language   Serbo-Croat
Religion   Muslim, Christian
Currency   Dinar

Sarajevo interviews

Two members of the Art Therapy Initiative visited Sarajevo from 5 to 9 May 1994 on behalf of War Child. Research in Sarajevo was restricted by the situation there at the time, and ATI members were limited by a five-day visiting permit. This blue card was at the time a compulsory document for entering and leaving the city. This was issued by UNHCR making access to the city possible. It was fortuitous that organisations were able to meet within these five days. In addition to the meetings referred to in Table 1, ATI was able to gain a comprehensive picture of the city by walking around the city, gaining insight into the functioning of Sarajevo at this time. They saw the frequently reported market-place which suffered two bombings, the old Muslim market, the Art Academy, the Holiday Inn, the UNHCR headquarters, the ruins of the Muslim Library.

Organisations interviewed	Existing psychological support for children and adults	Existing support for carers	Existing art or art therapy projects	Response to art therapy proposal in this context	Possibility of setting up a working structure	Could art therapy provide a service that was not already offered?
UNHCR	Support of orphanages and refugee centres: home visits to families in need	None known	None known	Positive: referred ATI to IRC for information on existing psychological support	Long-term: art therapy work in orphanages and refugee centres	Yes, in the long term; main focus of UNHCR on primary needs at this stage
IRC	Counselling bureau in 6 centres, 30 counsellors offering support to various sections of the community	Supervision and basic training for counsellors by IRC clinical psychologist	Knitting project: project for sale of handicrafts and art-works made by displaced people; art used in counselling as a diagnostic tool	Saw art therapy as fitting into and adding to existing IRC services	Immediate art therapy training for counsellors; longer-term: art therapy and referral system for families and children in need	Yes, training, art therapy and referral
UNICEF	Support primarily for children; psycho-social programme for traumatised children, art workshops, surveys to identify children at risk	Training and supervision; including programme of seminars of professionals, manuals and video-audio-tapes	Art workshops 'Step-by-Step to Recovery Programme'* in 10 primary schools; future plans to use art techniques for screening children for PTSD	Saw art therapy as useful	None proposed at this stage	Perceived their art workshops as already offering art activities seen as therapeutic
Others			A number of small international art projects planned to enhance the cultural life of the city			

***Table 1.** The psychological services in Sarajevo, May 1994*

This table depicts the depleted psychological services in Sarajevo at that time. The information was collected in May 1994 in a situation of war in which there was no centralised information and within the time-limits of ATI's visit. It is therefore not comprehensive.

Overall throughout this short period of time the following points were clear:
- The city had become isolated and both welcomed and needed outside support.
- The draining of professionals was sorely felt, leaving unrealistic demands on local untrained individuals working in the city. Appropriate training was unanimously perceived as essential, with art therapy contributing to this.†
- In response to ATI's research into the validity of War Child's proposal for an 'arts-based trauma centre' in Sarajevo, organisations saw this as an opportunity to draw together ideas and work already recognised as essential for their city and its people, over and above the stated long-term intentions of War Child. The different

*Appendix 2.
†See Conclusion to the research.

organisations interviewed perceived an immediate use for the centre as an information base for the different humanitarian aid work going on in the city.
- Although art therapy was virtually unknown in the city the organisations interviewed saw this as not only fitting in well into their already existing work but also as contributing a valuable and pertinent expertise to this situation.

East Mostar interviews

Two members of the Art Therapy Initiative visited East Mostar from 12 to 17 October 1994 on behalf of War Child.

The aim was to research the possibility of setting up an *arts-based trauma centre* in East Mostar (in the bombed music school), with art therapy integral to this. By this date, the city was divided with the east occupied predominantly by Bosnian Muslims and the west predominantly by Bosnian Croats. Since ATI's research in Sarajevo, War Child had established the charity in East Mostar and had set up its mobile bakery which produced 2000 loaves of bread each day for the city. The city was on orange alert* as a result of renewed shelling; despite this, ATI was able to meet with a number of organisations and individuals (Table 2).

The painting of the water tank at the War Child Bakery made available to the war child workers and their children the materials and structure for a few hours of art-making in their environment. It also provided ATI with an informal opportunity to make contact with twenty children and their parents (bakery workers) through art (Figs. 2 and 3., Pl. 1). This was important as it was impossible and premature to start art therapy while the war continued and was something ATI could offer in this context; to observe a response to art in a small way. Everybody participated and the atmosphere was spirited: this was the first time in three weeks that these parents and children had gathered in a group. The materials used were spray and car-paints. The painting expressed a personal relationship to their city and recent experiences: to the old bridge (now lost), river and houses.

The response to the art-making was important for ATI to observe as this would hold indications for art therapy work in the future. Whether the response had a tendency to be a constructive and contained expression, or a destructive and unboundaried one, as art therapists ATI had a responsibility to contain that which arose. The painting was contained and provided a few hours of creativity and fun.

---

*'Orange alert' means that children and adults cannot gather in groups, such as school.

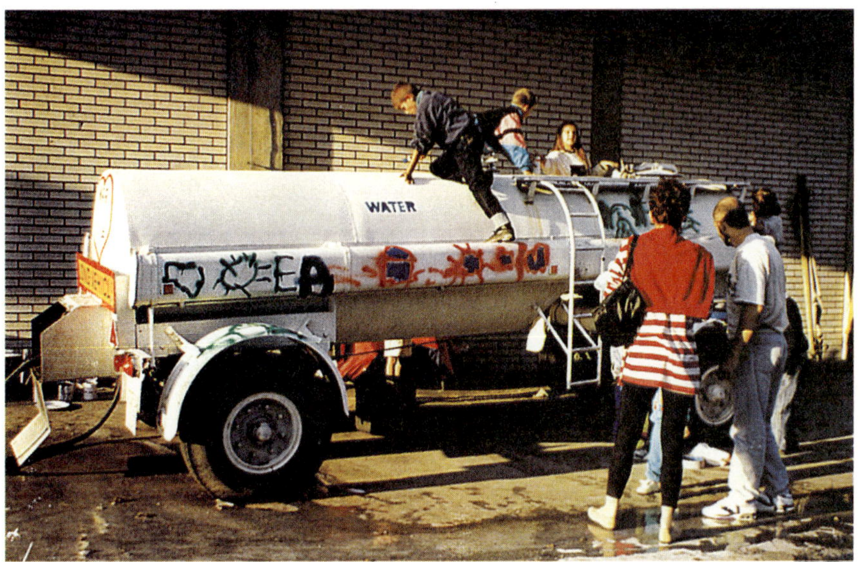

Fig. 2. Children painting the War Child water tank as parents look on. The tank was painted in a group at the War Child bakery in East Mostar.

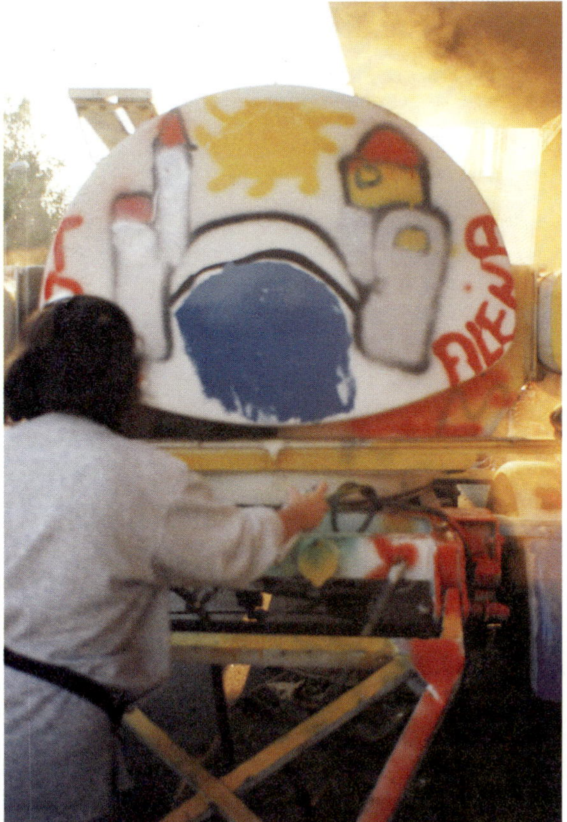

Fig. 3. The Mostar bridge (before the war) painted on one end of the War Child water tank. The tank was painted in a group at the War Child bakery in East Mostar.

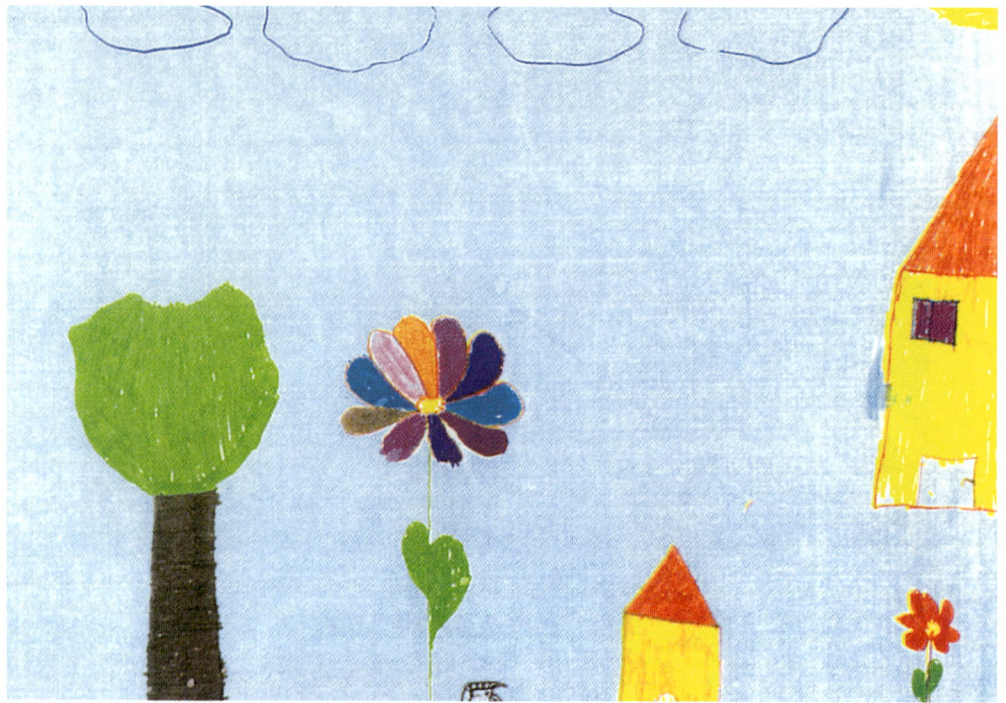

Fig. 6. House drawn by a 9-year-old girl in a group art session, Hrastnik refugee centre

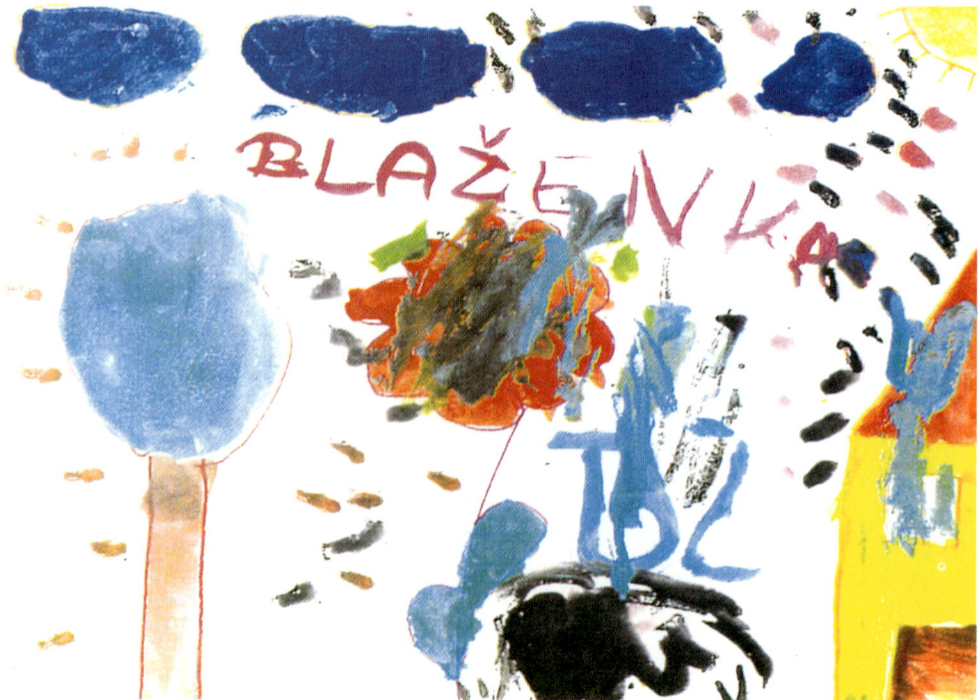

Fig. 7. House painted by the same 9-year-old girl (who painted fig.6) in the same art session, 20 minutes later, Hrastnik refugee centre

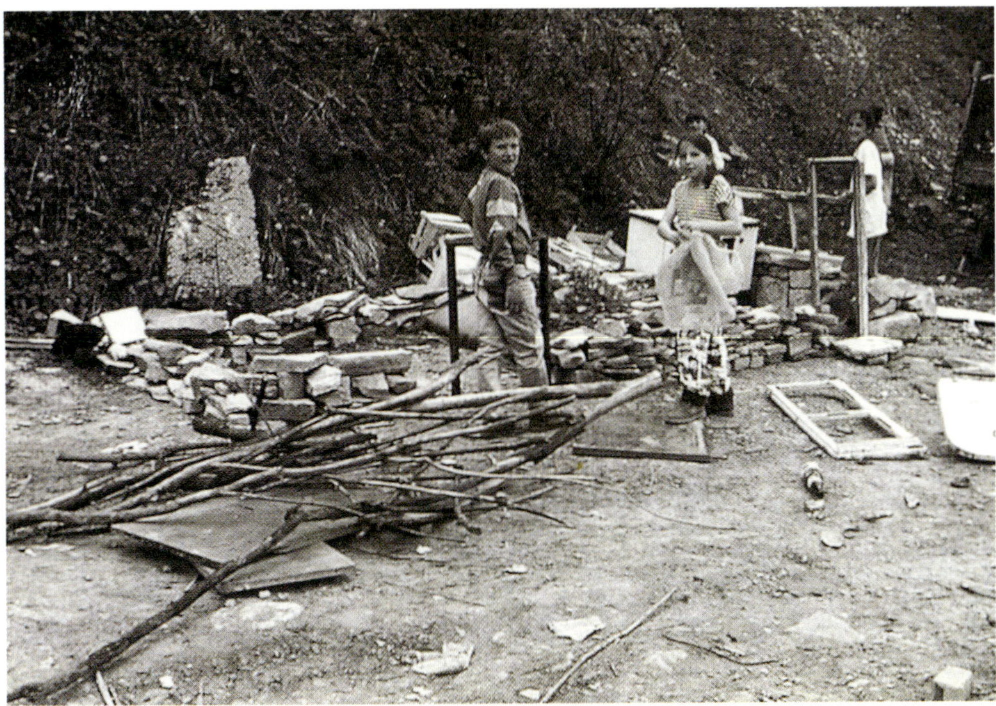

Fig. 8. Children make a home in the town dump,
Hrastnik refugee centre

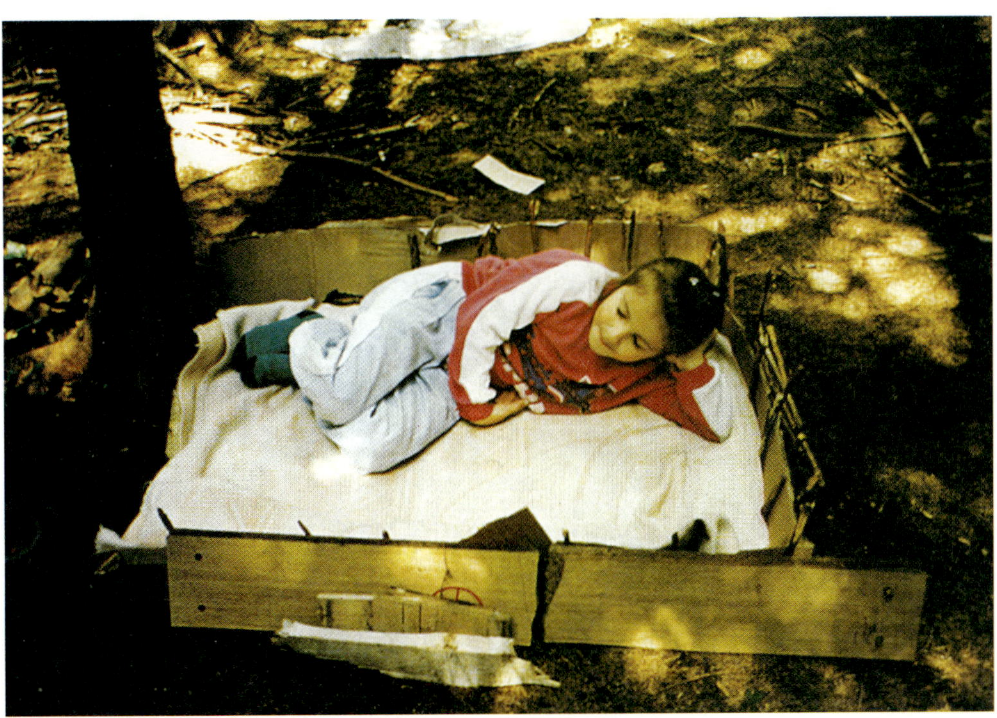

Fig. 9. Child makes a home in the woods,
Hrastnik refugee centre

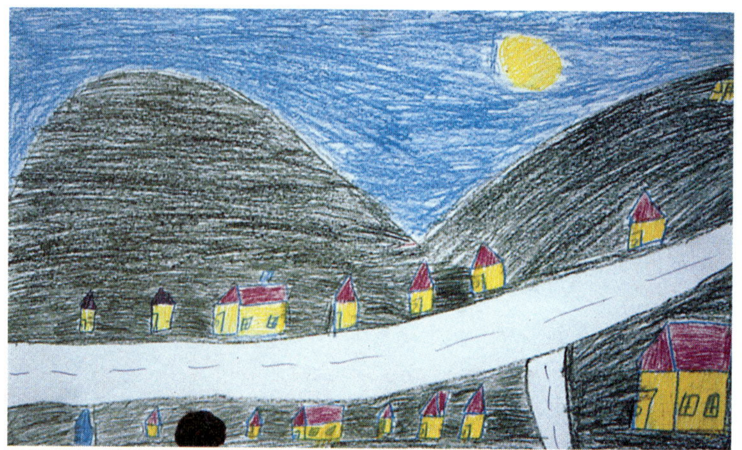

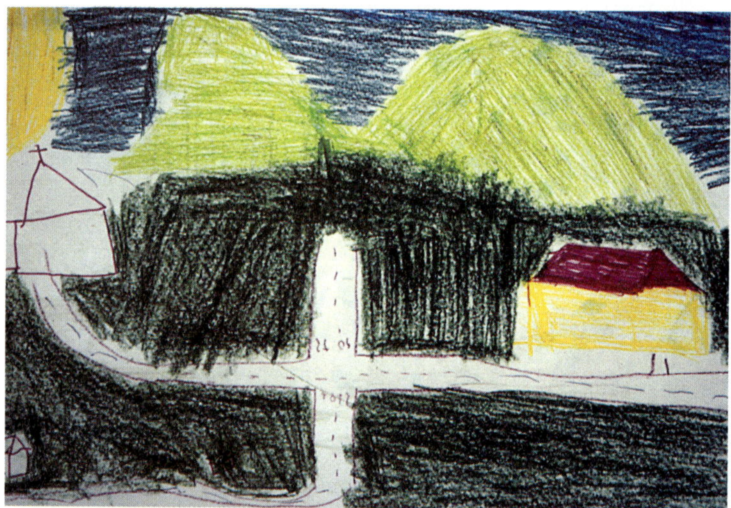

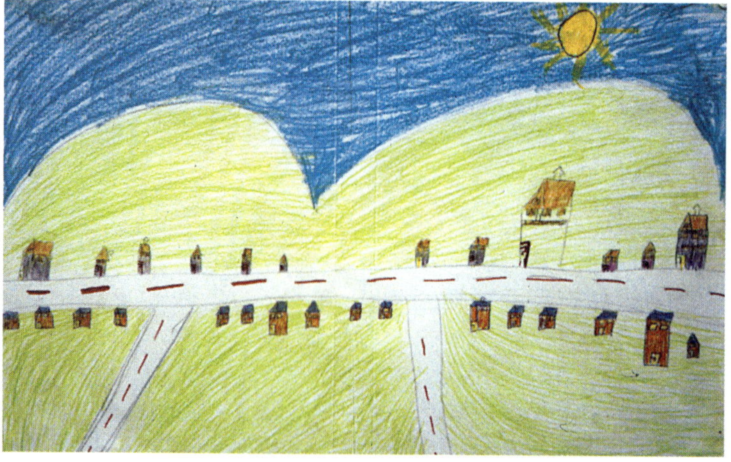

Fig. 13 – 15. **Roads or paths drawn by three different individuals, Prvic refugee centre**

Organisations interviewed	Existing psychological support for children and adults	Existing support for carers	Existing art or art therapy projects	Response to art therapy proposal in this context	Possibility of setting up a working structure	Could art therapy provide a service that was not already offered?
Omladinski Centre	Youth centre working with children and adolescents; discussion groups; irregular support from UNICEF psychologist	Not applicable	Two-month summer programme run by Italian organisation ICS, using music, speech, drawing, writing, etc.	Positive: seen as compatible with, and adding to, future plans	Long-term: art therapy can be implemented within the centre's working structure	Yes, training, art therapy and referral
Kindergartens	Intermittent support from UNICEF psychologists for children and parents	None	Art activities as part of school day; short ICS programme using mostly play	Art therapy seen as extremely valuable only if input is to be consistent	Yes, within the working structure of the 7 kindergartens	Yes, art therapy for children and, where appropriate, art therapy for parents and families
Zalic Centre (Orphanage)	Support for children provided by clinical psychologist	None	None, except informal art-making	Art therapy seen as useful due to lack of professionals and in work with children difficult to reach emotionally	Yes, within the working structure of the orphanage	Yes, art therapy for children
Soros Foundation	Not applicable	Not applicable	None	Art therapy proposal seen as fulfilling criteria for much needed local psychological support	Soros discussed possibility of funding ATI to implement therapy within local structures	Yes
Other	Not possible to meet with all aid organisations contacted, understood that UNICEF (which also carried out survey to identify children at risk), Médecins sans Frontières and Marie Stopes offered some psychological support	Not known	Not known			

Table 2. **The psychological services in East Mostar, October 1994**

This table depicts the depleted psychological services in East Mostar at this time. The information was collected in October 1994 in a situation of war in which there was no centralised information and within the time-limits of the visit. It is therefore not comprehensive.

At the time of ATI's visit to East Mostar, most resources were destroyed and the majority of the professionals had left the city. All those ATI met with expressed their need to accept whatever was offered from any source and the urgency to reconnect with the international world. At this time, there was little psychological support in East Mostar. UNICEF had plans to develop psychological services in each school in the city. Because teachers had often worked with the same children for several years before the war, UNICEF planned to train these teachers in counselling work.

ATI found the following: there was widespread alcoholism; often two families shared one or two rooms; individuality, personality, choice, privacy were often denied; there was little connection between parents and adolescents; help within the families was limited; bereavement was widespread; everybody lived with war daily. It was therefore clear that War Child's idea to establish an 'arts-based trauma centre' was well-founded as the need and desire for psychological support was, as has been demonstrated, fundamental.

ATI found that art projects have a positive role to play in providing a creative outlet. These are effective as a result of clear boundaries: limited and achievable time-frame, e.g. two hours or one day; the art project could be completed without need for follow-up.

Art therapy in the context of continuing war was not possible as individuals were daily re-experiencing the traumatic events of the war and needed to hold on to their coping strategies. Once the war was over and the situation for individuals was more stable, art therapy could contribute a valuable and pertinent expertise to the post-war services in East Mostar.

Croatia report

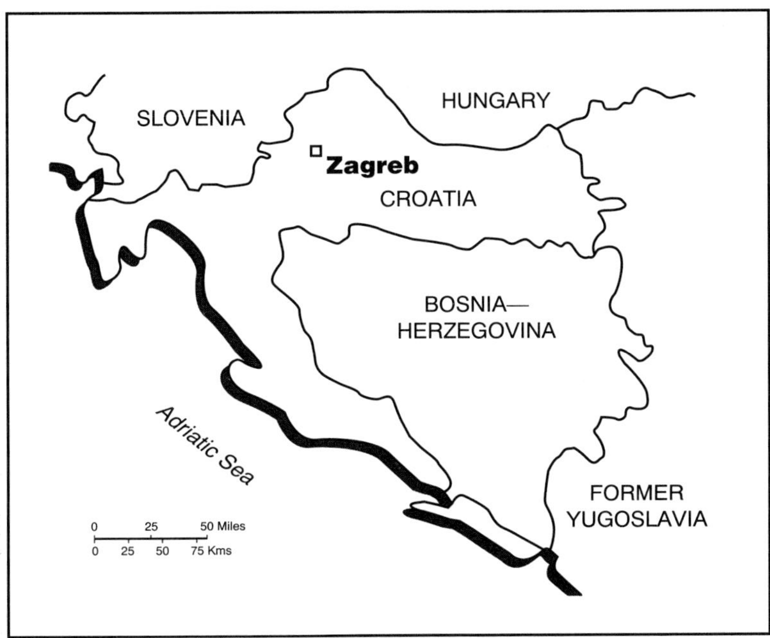

Figure 4. **Map of Croatia, 1996**

The Republic of Croatia

Status	Republic
Area	56,540 sq km (21,825 sq miles)
Population	4,511,000
Capital	Zagreb
Language	Serbo-Croat
Religion	Roman Catholic majority
Currency	Kuna
Organisations	UN

Zagreb interviews

Two members of ATI met with the following organisations in Zagreb on behalf of Goldsmiths' College, London University, on 3 and 4 October 1994. The aim was to reconnect with links that had already been made before the war between the Art Psychotherapy Unit at Goldsmiths' College and psychological services in Croatia. These links had been put in abeyance as a result of the war. ATI also aimed to gather information on psychological services available in the city and was able to meet with five individuals and organisations based in Zagreb. The overall intention was to see where art therapy could fit into the services already in place in Zagreb and/or Croatia at large.

Croatia at this time had not been involved in direct war since 1992 and was experiencing relative stability. A recurring theme in all the meetings was that there was a desperate lack of professionals and an immense need. All the professionals with whom ATI spoke were themselves suffering 'burn-out' and feeling overwhelmed by the need and the reality of numbers of individuals experiencing post-war problems: not only were local Croatians reacting to the experiences of the war, but there was an increasing influx of 'traumatised' refugees into Croatia, largely from Bosnia. In addition, many Croatian people had fled their villages before the war and were now unable to return as their villages had been destroyed, leaving them displaced. Many places throughout Croatia, such as Slavonski Brod in the north-east, had experienced shelling, heavy raids and casualties and had been neglected due to difficulties of physical access and lack of professionals. Besides the problems outlined above, the war had created additional problems: psychiatric wards destroyed leaving patients uncared for; widespread alcohol and behavioural problems amongst refugees and local people with inadequate support for these.

All the professionals felt a need for a break from their daily war-related work-loads and a desire to get back to pre-war interests and areas of expertise, e.g. working with eating disorders. The overall response to art therapy work was one of hope, not only as it was seen that art would be an appropriate tool for working with war-related issues, but art therapy would also add to the sorely depleted services available. Despite this, in all interviews, the lack of funding was raised and it was clear that this project could only work with independent funds.

Research interviews (Table 3) provided ATI with essential information into the context of Zagreb and an introduction to Croatia in general. They also provided a window into the potential for the use of art therapy both short and long term. The majority were already familiar with the discipline of art therapy and were interested to implement this as part of their psychological services, perhaps in Zagreb but most urgently in the neglected small towns of Croatia. Despite this, however, funding always proved to be a stumbling block.

Organisations and individuals interviewed	Existing psychological support for children and adults	Existing support for carers	Existing art or art therapy projects	Response to art therapy proposal in this context	Possibility of setting up a working structure	Could art therapy provide a service that was not already offered?
Luna film	Programme using film, specifically for gifted children who have experienced trauma	None known	Yes, using film	Interested in the discipline of art therapy in relation to a belief in art as a method of working with trauma	None at this stage	Yes
B–H Woman	Working mainly with women offering a work therapy scheme supported by a psychiatrist and general practitioner	Limited	Work therapy knitting project	Art therapy seen as appropriate for women and children and also as holding the potential for filling an urgent need for additional psychological support	To support the women using B–H Woman's services in Zagreb and to begin immediate work with their children	Yes
Zagreb Children's Hospital	Responsible for centralising psychiatric support for children affected by the war, including different therapies; serious shortage of professionals	Severely lacking	None	Short-term therapy and long-term training seen as useful	Short-term art therapy for children to be implemented immediately. Long-term therapy for children to be organised and training for local professionals established	Yes
Dr Sarajlich, Refugee camps in Varazdin, Croatia	Team of psychologists to train lay counsellors to serve the refugees in the camps	Details not known, lay counsellors received supervision and training from psychologists. Peer supervision amongst lay counsellors also in place	None. Photography used in counselling	Positive; art therapy perceived as adding to limited services in place	Not discussed in detail as funding unavailable	Yes
Clinic for psychological medicine, Rebro	Psychotherapy for children and adults	Not known	Art used in psychotherapy with children	Positive; art therapy and training seen as necessary	Various possibilities for setting up working structures in different settings	Yes

Table 3. **Information from meetings in Zagreb, October 1994**

This table depicts the information gathered from meetings held in Zagreb on 3 and 4 October 1994. The information is not comprehensive as time was limited. The overwhelming problems resulting from the war: the needs of local people, displaced people and refugees, the lack of professionals in Zagreb and Croatia overall at this time were emphasised in every meeting.

Split interviews

Two members of the Art Therapy Initiative met with international aid organisations involved in psycho-social work in Split in October 1994. Split had been a thriving tourist and holiday centre before the war and although at this time life in the city was returning to a semblance of normality there were still clear signs of the unresolved conflict. Most of the hotels were occupied by refugees and UN trucks constantly passed along the main road into and out of Bosnia. Besides the local people, the city was populated by refugees, displaced people and international aid workers.

Organisations and individuals interviewed	Existing psychological support for children and adults	Existing support for carers	Existing art or art therapy projects	Response to art therapy proposal in this context	Possibility of setting up a working structure	Could art therapy provide a service that was not already offered?
Save the Children	None	Not known	None	Saw art therapy as useful for pre-school children in schools	Art therapists could offer training to teachers in the sensitive use of art in their work in addition to art therapy with pre-school children	Yes
Marie Stopes International	Counselling groups for women with a view to self-help	Training for lay counsellors, also serving as support for this group of women	Art is used informally, resulting in thematic exhibitions, lack of training identified	Art therapy could have a valuable input	Valuable long-term input, mostly to train community workers in the sensitive use of art; also for support/art therapy for lay counsellors	Yes
Social Services UNHCR, Split	Responsible for all refugee and displaced people in Split and along the Dalmatian Coast, offering psychological support to children and adults although serious lack of professionals	Limited	Informal art-making; no art therapy	Interested to consider incorporating art therapy into UNHCR's psychological programme	Stable environment along the Dalmatian Coast conducive to art therapy	Yes
American Refugee Committee (ARC)	Responsible for psycho-social work in several refugee centres in Croatia: see 'Refugee centres in Croatia'	Supervision for psychologists	None	Art therapy seen as relevant to ARC's psycho-social programme	Yes, within existing ARC psycho-social service; see 'Refugee centres in Croatia'	Yes

Table 4. Services in Split and along the Dalmatian Cost, October 1994

This table provides a picture of services in Split and along the Dalmatian Coast at this time. The information was gathered from interviews held with international aid organisations in Split from 7 to 10 October 1994. As meetings were difficult to set up, information is not comprehensive.

The organisations listed in Table 4 provided ATI with information relevant to this research and contributed crucial background information to the context of Split at this time. All could envisage art therapy as contributing to the services they already offered but were however limited by funds at this stage.

Refugee centres in Croatia

Two members of the Art Therapy Initiative met with ARC, American Refugee Committee, between 20 October and 8 November 1994. ARC was responsible for psycho-social work in several refugee centres in Croatia. As previously mentioned, the influx of refugees into Croatia was presenting a large problem for the authorities throughout the country, in terms of housing, integration, finance. Although now refugees by status, the backgrounds of individuals were diverse, with some coming from rural communities and others from large cities. Indeed, each refugee centre was markedly different due to: location; size of centre; quality and type of accommodation; level of integration into its local community; origin of refugees (for instance a concentration of refugees from cities or rural areas); level of financial support. In addition, some of the centres also accommodated displaced people from Croatia which presented another complexity. What was shared by all the centres was that they were predominantly populated by women and children who had lost their homes, members of their family, livelihoods. All were living in an extended state of not-knowing.

It would seem that art therapy could play a useful role as part of ARC's psychological services in many of their centres, as these were relatively stable both in terms of population and distance from the war.

Refugee centres	Existing psychological support for children and adults	Existing support for carers	Existing art or art therapy projects	Response to art therapy proposal in this context	Possibility of setting up a working structure	Could art therapy provide a service that was not already offered?
Bosnian Old People's Home, Vodice	A psychologist and social worker	None	None	Not applicable	Not applicable	Not applicable
Obanjan Island refugee camp	2 psychologists provided by ARC	Not known	None	Not suitable for art therapy	Not applicable	Yes, but not applicable
Hydro-Electra refugee camp	2 psychologists and a teacher working with pre-school children	Not known	None	Seen as immediately applicable	The existing structure would accommodate the setting up of an art therapy working structure and allow for a follow-up service	Yes
Ciovo private accommodation	2 teams provided by ARC: public health team for psychological support, working in 4 centres	Supervision groups offered to ARC staff	None	Both individual and group art therapy seen to serve a potentially useful role	The existing structure would accommodate the setting up of an art therapy working structure and allow for a follow-up service	Yes
Kastel Kambelovac	One psychologist and public health medical technicians	Not known	None	Individual and group art therapy seen as relevant	The existing structure would accommodate the setting up of an art therapy working structure and allow for a follow-up service	Yes

Table 5. **Refugee centres in Croatia, October–November 1994**

This table provides a picture of the existing psychological support provided by ARC in five refugee centres along the Dalmatian Coast. This information was gathered during visits made with ARC to the refugee centres between 20 October and 8 November 1994. The response and applicability of art therapy to this context was positive and evident in the table.

Pilot art therapy projects

Prvic, Croatia and Hrastnik, Slovenia

ATI carried out two pilot art therapy projects in the former Yugoslavia, the first of which took place at Hrastnik refugee centre in Slovenia (March–May, 1994 and August 1994) and the second at Prvic refugee centre (October–November 1994), on Prvic Island, situated off the Dalmatian Coast in Croatia. The overall aim of both pilot art therapy projects was to bring art to the refugee centres and to assess if/how art therapy could be used in the long term in these contexts. The two reports are presented in different styles, reflecting the two different forms the pilot projects took. In both situations, ATI members lived and worked in the refugee centres. The reports include descriptions of the art and art sessions as well as general experiences and perceptions of living in the camps. In documenting this, it is almost impossible, perhaps not useful, to separate one from the other.

Hrastnik refugee centre (Slovenia)

This report is written in a descriptive format. This was ATI's first visit to the former Yugoslavia and the visit was primarily exploratory with the variables largely unknown. As a result of this the structure of the art sessions developed organically. The aim of this visit (over and above the introduction of the art and assessment of the potential for art therapy) was to observe, informally, the life and the environment of the refugee centre so as to gain some small understanding of the experience of the people who found themselves refugees.

This project was initiated by ATI and supported by private sponsors, War Child and the Bosnian Support Group. The latter supports Hrastnik refugee centre by provision of volunteer workers, essential supplies and a family befriending scheme (with families in Great Britain pairing with families at Hrastnik refugee centre). The Bosnian Support Group was keen to add a therapeutic component to the aid they already provided. They saw art therapy as the most appropriate form of therapy for this centre and therefore supported ATI with the pilot project with a view to long-term implementation.

Prvic refugee centre (Croatia)

This report is written primarily in the form of a diary so as to retain as much detail as possible. This pilot project was more consciously structured, built upon, and informed by, the experience gained from the work at Hrastnik. This report is more formal in the sense that by now ATI was able to *think* more formally and reflectively upon their experience and the experience of the refugees. Although there was still much to learn, and much remained new and unknown, ATI had a greater awareness of the context in which they were working. Because the use of art had proved appropriate and beneficial in Hrastnik, ATI was able to introduce an informed art therapy structure, adapted to the daily routine of Prvic refugee centre.

The aim of this pilot project, over and above the introduction of the art and assessment of the potential for art therapy, was to increase ATI's understanding of art therapy work in the context of this war, and to adapt general art therapy knowledge to specific situations. Prvic refugee centre was identified by UNHCR as suitable for ATI's pilot project as it would benefit from additional support and employed a psychologist and social worker, part time, who could maintain follow-up support where needed.

The pilot art therapy project was initiated by ATI and supported by private sponsors and UNHCR, Split (Social Services). Misco Mimico, in his capacity as Head of Social Services, was responsible for the psychological support of the refugees and displaced populations in Split and along the Dalmatian Coast. Mr Mimico spoke of the severe lack of psychologists and caring professionals in his service at this time. As a result of this these professionals were spread thinly over many refugee centres and a wide area, often with one psychologist in charge of two or three centres. Mr Mimico was interested in ATI's proposal for art therapy as he saw this as potentially contributing to the Social Services support already in place. Mr Mimico envisaged that art therapy could perhaps take the form of an itinerant service, with art therapists working in more than one centre. He was interested to monitor the progress of the pilot project and requested a report at its completion.

Hrastnik refugee centre

Introduction

Slovenia gained independence from Yugoslavia in June 1991 after a short-lived conflict. Slovenia was able to divorce itself from the tragic events elsewhere in the former Yugoslavia, mainly because it does not have the same ethnic diversity as in other republics; 90 per cent of the population being Slovene.

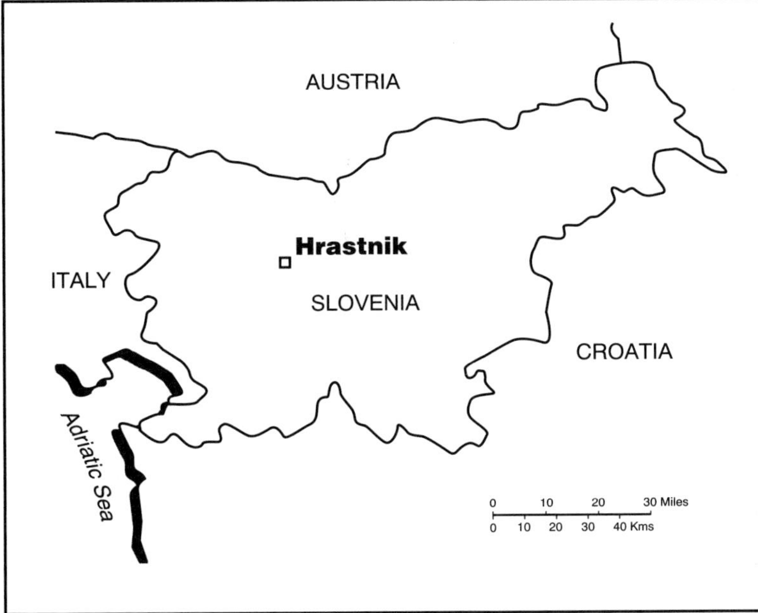

Figure 5. **Map of Slovenia, 1996**

Hrastnik is the largest coal-mining town in Slovenia, 40 miles from the capital of Ljubljana. The town is itself industrialised and is surrounded by hills and pine forests. The camp is set on the hillside on the edge of the town.

The refugee centre
Hrastnik refugee centre is surrounded by beautiful hillside, and flourishing allotments, belonging to local people. Although the allotments are in touching distance, the refugees had no access to them. The camp is 250 yards long and the six single-storey wooden huts that make up the camp are closely grouped on a dirt patch. On a summer's day, the place was bright with activity. On a dull day, it was reminiscent of a prison camp. The Slovenian government was responsible for the camp, employing a small team of local Slovenians to manage it. Six migrant workers' huts were allocated to the refugees, leaving one building for the immigrant Bosnian mineworkers who had been working there when the war started. The Swiss Disaster Relief Unit provided an all-purpose building, serving as the kitchen, dining room and school room. There were only four toilets and showers for the 200 refugees, and hot water for three hours each day.

The refugees
Initially refugees arrived from Bosnia in April 1992, and it was thought they would move back home after a few weeks. Two years later (May 1994), most of the two hundred people who fled their homes were still living in the camp on the hillside. Of these 107 were children, 72 were women and the remainder men. The refugees were allowed no freedom of movement, requiring passes to go even the ten minutes' walk into town. Everybody – refugees and staff – was faced with the bleak and real possibility that they may be there for a very long time to come.

In practice, the women took charge of the day-to-day routine, and there were too few men to make any real impact. The absent men were either dead or fighting, or their whereabouts unknown. Most of the men in the camp were either over sixty years of age, or were migrant workers before the war and had no official refugee status. The young men living in the camp were not regarded with much favour by those women who daily faced the reality that their husbands were not with them because they stayed to fight.

The children attended school in the all-purpose building which was divided in the middle by a blackboard at lesson times, enabling two classes to take place simultaneously, and then cleared away for meals. There were six unpaid teachers who were all refugees living at Hrastnik Camp. Four worked full-time and were unqualified. The two part-time teachers taught geography and English and were qualified in their subjects. The starting age for children was 8 years; there were 50 in the 8–12-year age group, 50 in the 13–18-year age group and 12 others with the ages 18–25 who attended no school. In addition to school, the permanent volunteer, Bernard McMahon, provided some classes, such as drawing with felt-tips for 4–8-year-olds, and a special English class for keen students. He was also attempting to set up a social club for 15 adolescents whom he had identified as needing additional support.

Psychological support
There was no formalised psychological support based at Hrastnik refugee centre. In 1993, a Spanish psychologist visited the centre for a period of three weeks and offered a variety of social, sport and educational activities. It was as a result of the lack of

psychological support that the Bosnian Support Group supported ATI's visit. The members of ATI lived in one of the six barracks with 35 others, in a room of their own that functioned as living space, bedroom and art therapy room.

The volunteers
The Bosnian Support Group provided the permanent volunteer. He had lived in the centre since 1993 and offered round-the-clock friendship, listening, and practical support. Additional volunteers were sent for shorter periods by the Bosnian Support Group to offer general support.

Art therapy at Hrastnik: Visit One

On arrival, the intention of ATI was to live in the refugee centre and gradually introduce art in to the structures already in place. However, the moment the refugees heard of the arrival of two artists, ATI were plunged into work and initiated a programme of art sessions earlier than they had anticipated. Apart from school, there was little else offered to either children or adults in the refugee centre.

There was a pervading atmosphere of boredom, weary anticipation and suppressed anger which was relieved by a brave humour, usually expressed over cups of sweet, thick Bosnian coffee, and a life of physical activity – scrubbing the corridors, adapting the room from bedroom to living space, washing the cooking implements, clothes, and the one shower shared by fifty others.

There was only one telephone, and whenever it rang, there was a period of suspense and a mass of activity around the office. On the evening of ATI's arrival in April 1994, the telephone rang for a mother of four with news of her husband's death by a grenade. Everyone was eating a supper of noodles at the time. The woman on the next table pushed her barely touched plate aside and sat with her head in her hands. At this stage, other families had heard no news about their fathers/husbands, and the Red Cross could not trace them.

Each room had a television dominating it, with the news channel turned on continuously giving Croatian news bulletins on the war. During daily morning coffee sessions, ATI listened to individual accounts and viewpoints of the war – as translated by Bernard.

By the second visit in August, news had come through that one man had been 'chopped to pieces' in a prison camp. Their neighbour had recently received better news: her husband made contact by the telephone in July, for the first time since the start of the war. He was well and still fighting and tried to call every few days. When he did not manage to, tensions rose and the waiting continued.

On this visit, ATI worked to make drawing and painting available to as many people as they could. Art took many forms as it was necessary to approach different age groups in different ways. Although most of the work focused on the children, ATI also held portrait classes for grandparents; evening embroidery groups for mothers; art lessons for teenagers. The 'mothers' would not come to an art session but were able to accept an embroidery class in the evenings (after the communal work was completed). Within this they were open to explore personal themes. (Embroidery is a traditional art form amongst this generation of Bosnian women.) In working with grandparents, art participation took the form of portrait drawing in which couples would spend the time looking at and drawing each other. Young people seemed to prefer groups in which themes such as drawing from still-life and portraiture were used as a starting point.

The children were by far the largest group in the camp and were therefore offered morning and afternoon art groups for up to 15 children. Houses soon emerged as the main theme. Most often children were encouraged to explore their own themes which usually resulted in an attempted drawing of the 'ideal' house (Fig. 6, Pl. 2). Sometimes the surfaces were marred (Fig. 7, Pl. 2) or unidentifiable objects would appear as if in spite of themselves, pieces would be gouged out of roofs, or the entire picture would be defaced or scribbled over – at times by another child.

The house theme led ATI to take a group of eight of the older children to a disused town dump where they built a house from the objects found. They unearthed an old stove, a washing basin, shelves, a bed, a sink, pots, pans, buckets, window-frames and by creating a human chain collected enough stones from a quarry to create the foundations of the building. The children took pride and delight in this house. When the house was knocked down by local children, the refugee children calmly reconstructed it as a group. Knocked down a second time, the children sat in the remains and made drawings of the house and the surrounding landscape. They also recorded the rubble using ATI's camera (Fig. 8, Pl. 3). Perhaps they wanted a permanent record, where no such record exists of their own destroyed homes.

The little children spontaneously made homes in the wood behind the camp. They collected bricks for chairs, wood for tables, flowers for decoration, sticks for demarcation. They even fetched blankets from their rooms, and climbed inside the marked-out spaces (Fig. 9, Pl. 3). Each day for a week other children knocked these houses down; each day they patiently rebuilt them.

Some of these children had spent long nights hiding in woods, before their arrival in Slovenia. All these 'homes' were vulnerable to attack, yet all had a marked-out skeleton of a boundary that suggested not only the need for containment, but also a fragility. Using a camera, the children were anxious to record the houses, standing and destroyed, placing themselves inside. It was powerful to observe both this act of destroying, and the patient and insistent recreating of what had been destroyed.

Art therapy at Hrastnik: Visit Two

The August visit lasted eight days. ATI returned to Hrastnik with Dr Nick Lessof, a paediatrician. On the first visit it became clear that no doctor had visited the camp for more than a couple of hours at a time and although the refugees had access to good medical care at the medical centre in Hrastnik, most found it quite an ordeal to make their way there, having to negotiate the half-hour walk, and then communicate in the Slovenian language. Others were too afraid to seek assistance for fear of what might be discovered about their health.

The aims of this visit were to re-make contact, to continue to provide emotional support and again provide an opportunity for the making of art in a formal setting. In addition, because the volunteers had by now lived and worked in the camp for several months at a time, their energies were depleted and ATI attempted to offer support by talking through issues that had arisen and exchanging ideas. One of the volunteers was encouraged to take a short break to enable her to re-stock her depleted energies and get a much earned and needed distance.

On the first visit a small activities hut had begun to be built and was now completed. Although this hut was funded by an Italian organisation, this was seen as an enormous development in that the Slovenian authorities were acknowledging the need for such activities. Art sessions could therefore take place in this room and not in the barracks. Although ATI offered general art sessions, the main project was the group painting of a mural (with 20 children and one grandmother) on two walls of the activities hut. On this occasion various mothers requested formal family photographic portraits which they hoped to send back to Bosnia. This request turned into a formal session which was conducted with great ceremony by the families who dressed in their best clothes and adopted a formal pose and serious expression. Nobody in the camp had a camera and it seemed important that ATI was asked to document this event at this stage. Even though this session was not an art session as such, it seemed to be consistent with the ethos of ATI offering support.

The intention was for ATI to visit Hrastnik Camp at intervals and to build on the work already initiated, exploring with the refugees issues such as coping with loss, displacement, continuing uncertainty as to their future. A further visit had been planned for October 1994. This was however impossible to follow through due to the local situation in which the Slovenian authorities had instated a new clause in which additional foreign visitors were unable to visit Hrastnik refugee centre for more than a day at a time. Because of this, ATI has been unable to develop this work further.

ATI has, however, been able to maintain continuing contact with Hrastnik through the volunteers there and with the Bosnian Support Group in London. It is understood that, following the Peace Agreement in November 1995, families were beginning to make plans to return home, while some had already left. The Bosnian Support Group is continuing to support them on their return to Bosnia, funds permitting. Although the Slovenian Government is in the process of closing the camp down, some families intend to remain in the area permanently while others have joined members of their families in other host countries. (See Update 1996, page 63.)

Conclusion

The response to the art-making was surprising in its immediacy and was more successful than ATI could have envisaged. The initial premise was that the work would have to be tentative with a desire not to impose a model of art therapy which may not be applicable or welcome. ATI began from the premise however that art and art therapy would have a great deal to contribute. The intention was to begin with a period of observation and listening before introducing art. Almost at once however, they realised that what was expected was the immediate provision of a creative outlet, particularly for children. The refugee children seemed parched of any stimulus and the parents themselves seemed thirsty for input which would support them in helping their children.

ATI developed a style of work in response to the circumstances and the art sessions evolved over the period of five weeks. In addition to introducing a general art group each morning for children, ATI decided to offer an art therapy group for five children identified as in need of particular emotional support, which would meet at the same time each morning for the five weeks. The group was impossible to maintain however due to the established camp 'culture' of the refugees which was unwilling to readily accommodate an additional fixed time each day. The refugees were keen to organise their time as individually as the imposed timetable would allow. However, this particular group of children with whom ATI began to work became constant members of the general art groups throughout the five weeks of the first visit.

The answers to the initial hypotheses and questions ATI set out became apparent very quickly through working and living in the refugee centre environment. It was working with the answers found, adapting to the knowledge gained and remaining flexible which proved most informative. The following are examples of the themes which developed over the pilot art therapy project.*

Maps
Ed Vulliamy (1994), author of *Seasons in Hell: Understanding Bosnia's War,* described this war as the 'War of Maps' and the war of the *narod* (the Slavonic word resembling the German term *das Volk* and meaning 'people' and 'nation' at the same time):

> In the War of Maps and of the narod, there is no such thing as objective history, and no consensus over the maps that delineate the rightful frontiers of this narod or that. With what becomes either an irksome or terrifying tedium, history dominates every interview in the Bosnia War. The answer to a question about an artillery attack yesterday will begin in the year 925, invariably illustrated with maps. (Vulliamy, 1994, p. 5)

> In the middle of the War of Maps is Bosnia–Herzegovina. Over this country, the frontiers of Serbia or Croatia, and the wayward dreams of each, interweave, overlap and retreat down the centuries and into the proposed future. (Vulliamy, 1994, p. 10)

The first and only art therapy theme that ATI introduced at Hrastnik (into an already established group for young people which met one evening each week) was that of the map in its broadest sense. This was to be interpreted widely and was offered tentatively and with an awareness that this may raise many very personal responses which could be worked with over the five-week visit. A group of the young people decided to create a large map of Bosnia together. This took on a meaning that was significant to this group and to the majority of the refugees. The strength of response to this map was indeed surprising.

The map was moved from dining room to art room and back to dining room. Initially the young people who created it added their towns and villages; later, the children, and elder members of the community added their names and those of their children and grandchildren, so that in the end the map was a tapestry of names and personal histories (Figure 10). The map seemed therefore not only to provide a concrete vehicle for stating a personal history but also to serve on an emotional level in which families came together to make their mark and in some cases this allowed for silent moments

---

*The detailed documentation of obstacles to art therapy work and practical considerations can be found in 'Conclusion to research' at the end of Part II.

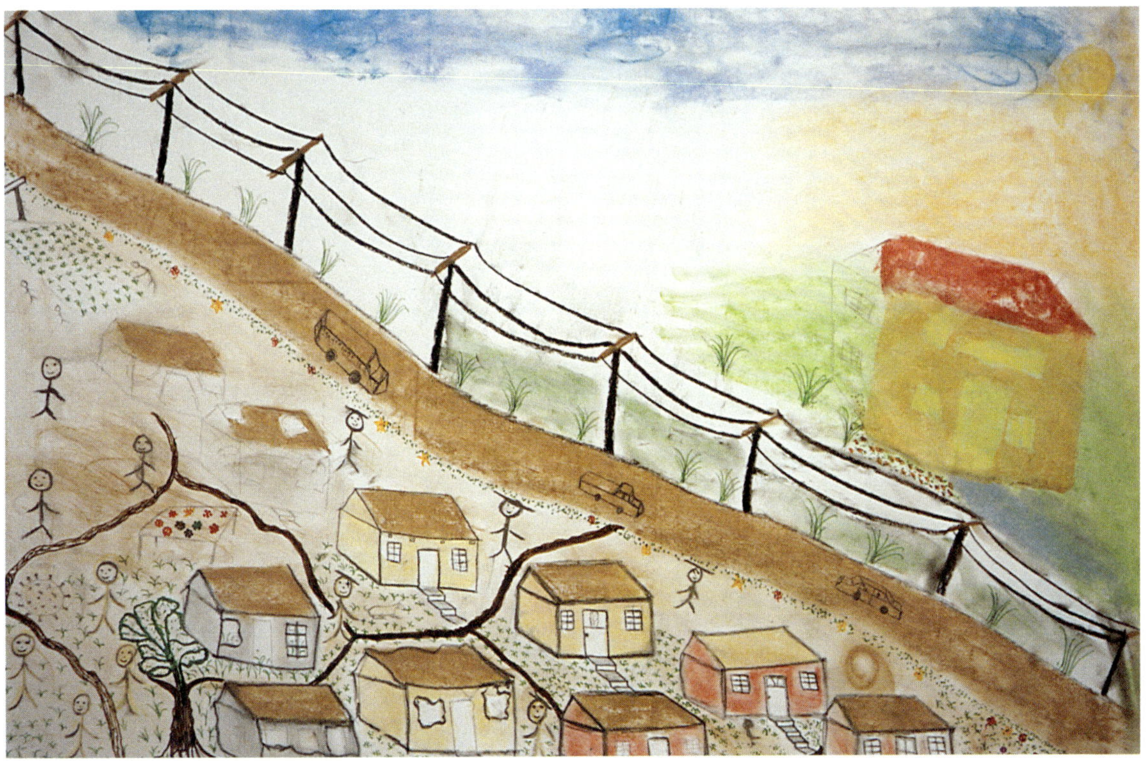

Fig. 18. **A road separating a black township from a white area.**
The township is full while the white area is incomplete. The artist did not complete the picture.
Drawing made in an open art therapy studio, KwaZulu–Natal, South Africa

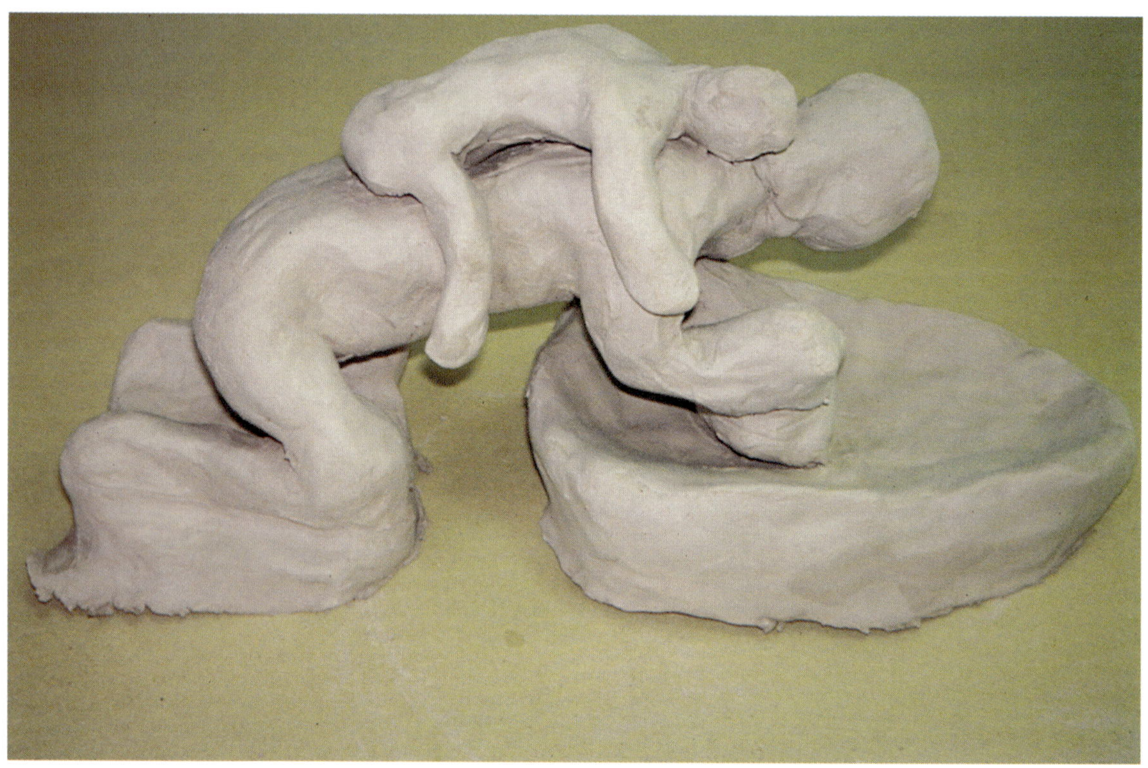

Fig. 19. **A woman doing washing with baby on back.**
Sculpture made in a materials workshop, KwaZulu–Natal, South Africa

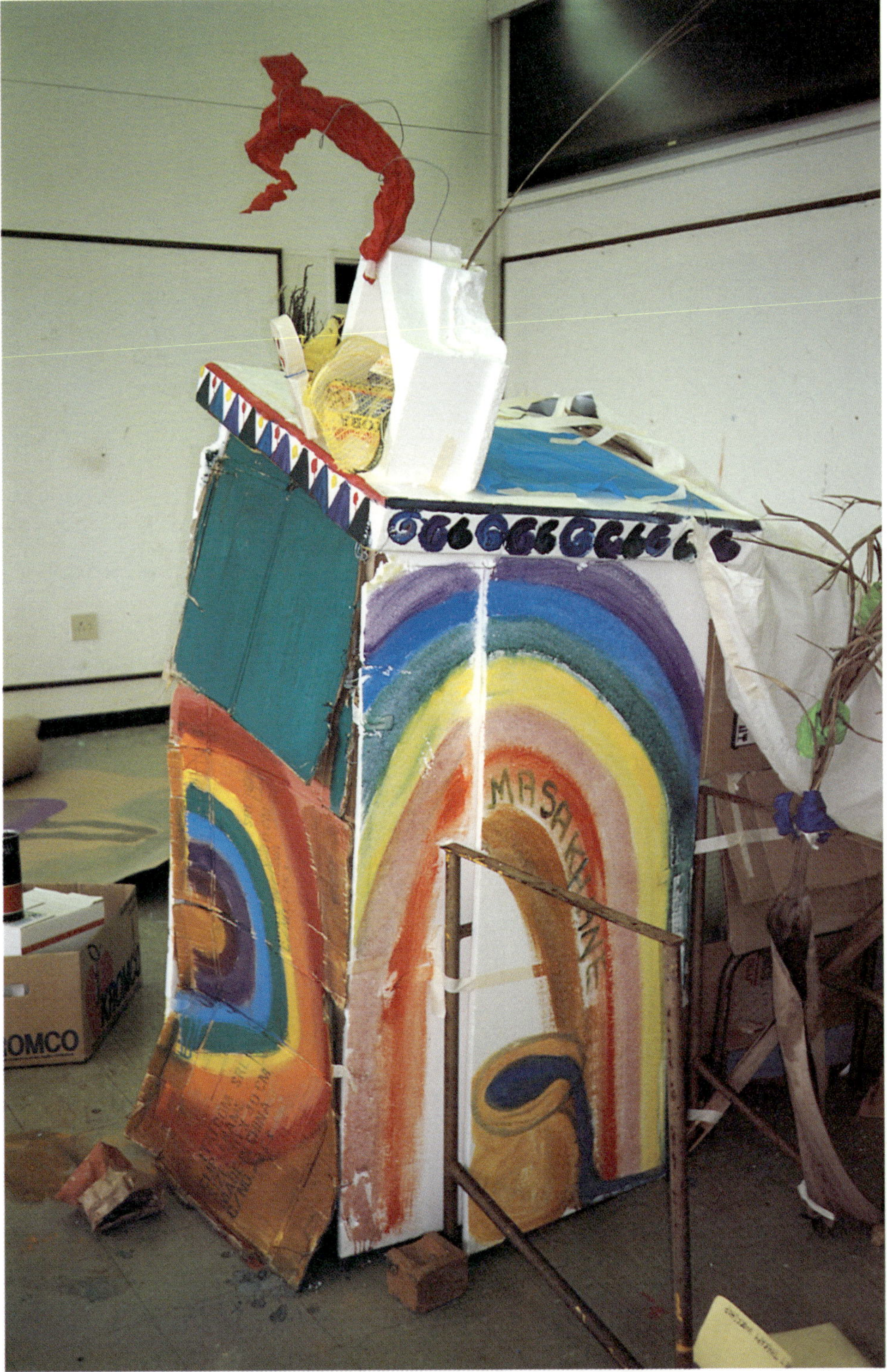

Fig. 20. This house was made out of scrap by the participants as a group.
Sculpture made in a theme workshop, KwaZulu–Natal, South Africa

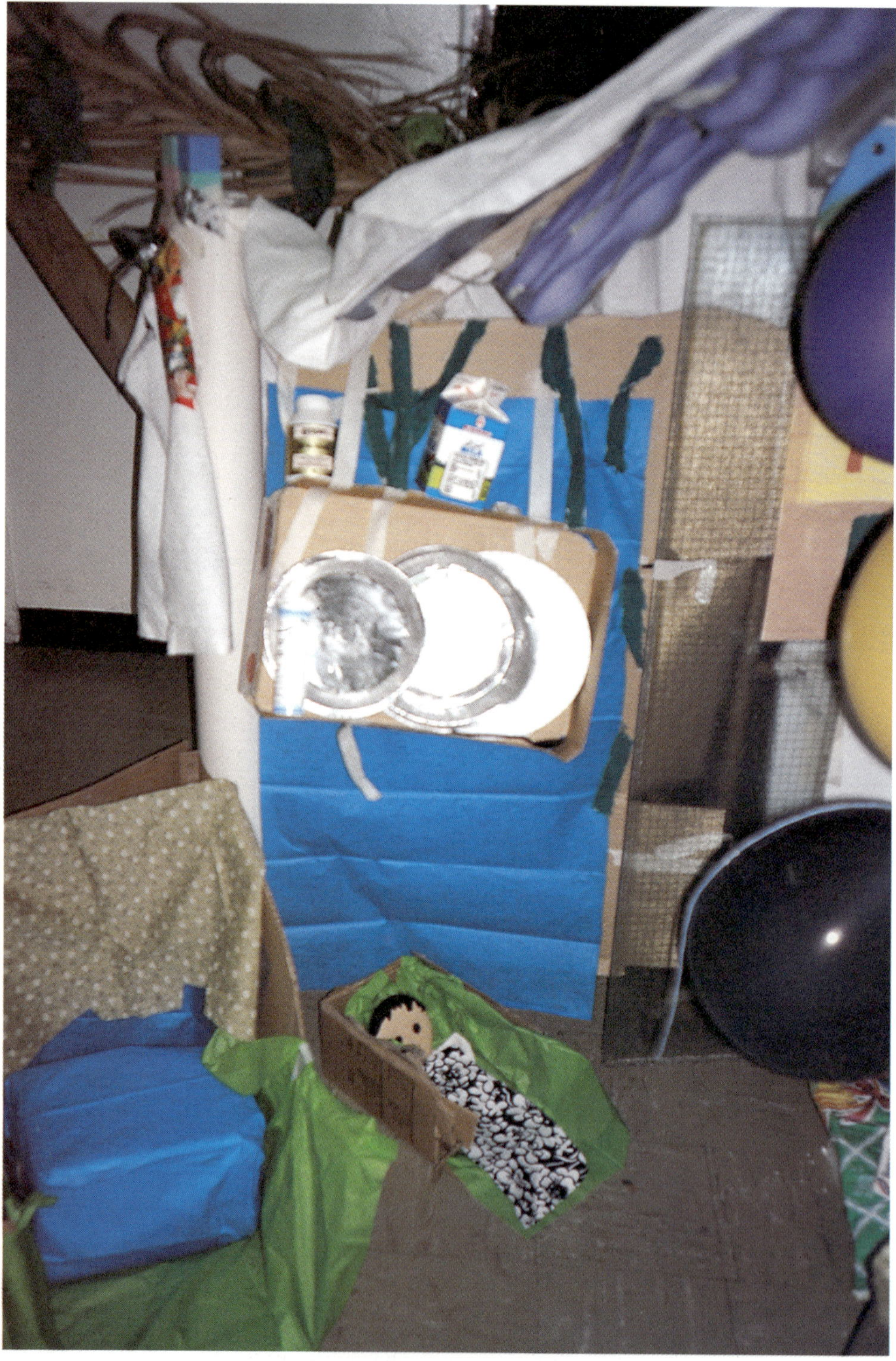

Fig. 21. ‘The inside of the house’ in Fig 20.
Sculpture made in a theme workshop, KwaZulu–Natal, South Africa

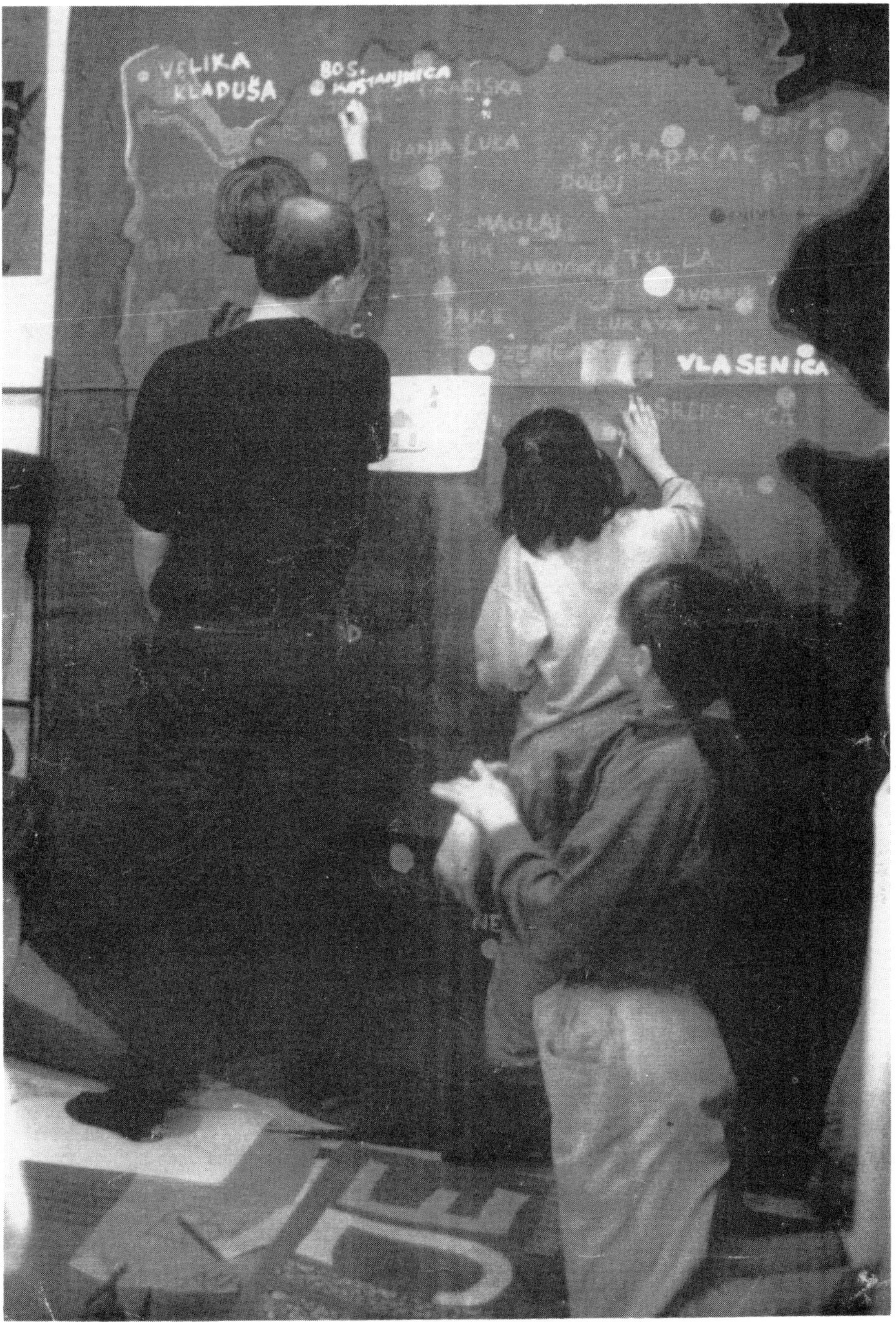

Figure 10. Children paint on their map of Bosnia, Hrastnik refugee centre

of grieving. As art therapists ATI were aware of the therapeutic value this work was offering: the theme allowed for a number of personal responses on different levels. For some it served as an unintrusive means for enabling personal grieving, for others it served as a vessel for placing themselves in a context, for others it provided a concrete statement of a collective loss, as well as expression of their individuality and pride in their history. The dehumanising reality of the war and being forced to become by identity 'refugees', had for these people, on a small level been challenged through the art . Individuals could express and show that they had not always been refugees placed in a refugee camp.

Houses
The depiction of houses was to evolve as a central theme in the art sessions and was to become an apparent preoccupation and a theme of some importance amongst children of all ages and in many art forms: drawing, building (as discussed in the report), story-telling and the staging of small dramas. This representation of houses continued over the five weeks, after ATI left and was still present on ATI's second visit to the camp.

There was little need to motivate the children who seemed to have their own momentum and need to express themselves. The art sessions offered children a facilitated vehicle for this expression which held more complexity than could perhaps be communicated verbally at that time. Through the art-making there was more space for metaphor, and as it moved away from the literal it was able to hold and contain different meanings and work on different levels. The houses could have meant a number of things: they perhaps provided the opportunity to re-enact a drama, survive and own it. Perhaps some of these children had been trying to visualise the damage done to their own homes, and had been impotent to change it. Through the process of making and re-making perhaps the children were beginning to come to terms with their desolation and loss. Perhaps this making over and over again – particularly for the younger children – suggested a re-enacting of the trauma which provided no relief and needed a form of intervention before this could happen. Perhaps the house appeared as it is a symbol that recurs throughout cultures and is a healthy part of all children's play. Over the span of the pilot project, issues such as ownership and authorship, finding one's own space and placing oneself inside it, became crucial and were usually resolved through the activity. It is hoped that the above work demonstrates the important role art can play in the context of this refugee camp in aiding the individuals in the process of coming to terms with their experience.

Prvic refugee centre

Introduction

Prvic is a small island situated off the Dalmatian Coast, near to Sibenik, Croatia. The population was at this time, about 300 – mostly elderly, with 50 children who attended the two local schools or schools in mainland Sibenik. Fifty years ago, there were nearly 5000 inhabitants but – as the island has been through two recent wars (there are still remnants of the Second World War in the form of a series of bunkers that sit on the hill above the refugee centre) – many people are now living in Croatia, Australia, the USA or Europe. The island had been a tourist centre before this latest war but it was to hard to imagine this as the island was now very quiet with two small villages, each with two shops and the only people visible were elderly, seated on benches during the late afternoon. Those going to the mainland or arriving at the island were transported by the two boats each day, which alternated their rota weekly. At the time ATI worked there, there was little sense of the war and life continued for the inhabitants, with octopus fishing and olive picking. The lack of visitors, however, and the presence of the refugee centre at the end of the smallest of the villages were daily proof of the recent conflict in Croatia and the continuing war in Bosnia.

During ATI's pilot project on Prvic from October to November 1994 there were marked changes in the island's weather from calm and quiet periods to strong winds and driving rain.

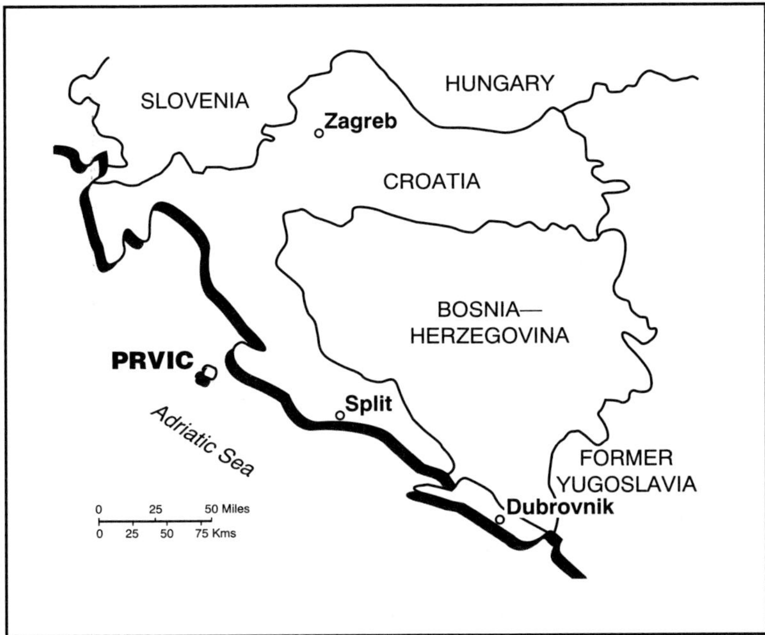

Figure 11. Map of Croatia, 1996

The refugee centre

The scout summer camp building which accommodated the refugee centre is situated in front of a small bay and at the foot of a hill covered with pine trees. It is a substantial square building built on three floors, large enough to house 70 people. At this time, as a refugee centre, there was a central dining/living room, a large kitchen and small office/first-aid room. Each floor held bedrooms providing bunk-beds, and two toilets. There were only two showers, situated on the ground floor. Outside is a patio area, a covered area which had tables in the summer, a yard for hanging-out washing, an area of rough grass, and a second paved area with two table tennis tables.

The centre was officially opened in October 1994, with visits by Misco Mimico, (Director of Social Services at UNHCR, Split), local newspapers and television. There were only 24 refugees in the centre when ATI arrived in late October. The centre was given over for refugees in June 1994, and it was converted by 'Care Canada' who put up partition walls for bedrooms. The Director of the centre was a Croatian man and secretary of 'Our Children' – a Croatian government organisation soon to become a humanitarian aid organisation. A nurse attended to emergency first-aid needs between 10 am and 4 pm, Monday to Saturday. Otherwise, the first-aid room was locked from four in the afternoon, until the following morning and in the case of an emergency or any first-aid need, the refugees would have to take the boat to go to the hospital on the mainland, where they would have to pay. Two cooks worked in shifts, preparing and serving the food, locking the kitchen when they left. One meal each day was supplied by the Red Cross in the form of standard tinned or processed rations.

The refugees
Most of the children at the centre were separated from their parents, who were either still in Bosnia, or had died in the war. There were 9 children between the ages of 2 and 11, a baby of 4 months, 11 adolescents, and 3 women. The initial criteria was for 'traumatised children without parents'. This soon shifted to 'children with one parent' but the criteria continued to evolve according to need.

The Office for Displaced People and Refugees (ODPR) was the only office in Croatia for people to acquire legal papers, and this centre on Prvic acted as an official address from which to make an application. As a result of this, the centre became a place of transition for people who came with no papers, and intended to move to other countries or return to Bosnia.

Refugees were reluctant to come to the centre as it is situated on an island and transportation is infrequent and difficult. The refugees had no personal income other than the small amount provided by the ODPR every three months, and the extra money made by making and selling clothes in the sewing workshop. Also, two Muslim organisations, Idasa and Merhamed, gave a small stipend.

The younger children, ages 6–11, attended the local schools on the island while the adolescents were required to attend school in Sibenik.

Psychological support
Psychological support was provided by two women who were responsible for liaising with Care Canada and the Director of the centre. For Natasa, a trained psychologist, and Mari, a teacher who acted as a social worker this was their first job. Both were also in charge of the psychological support at the Elderly Refugee Camp at Vodice.

The volunteers
There was a volunteer programme from Zagreb which provided volunteers from Europe (particularly Switzerland). The aim of the programme was to provide social and creative activities and to bring fresh input, support and friendship from outside, to reduce the sense of isolation of the refugees. Volunteers played an important role, but it was expected that there would be a difficulty in sustaining them during the University Terms.

The local population
The local population of about 300 people was mostly elderly, and had lived on the

island for generations. Although the original intention was to integrate the refugees into the local community, only five months had passed and already there was local antagonism and a desire for the refugees to leave the island. The refugee children however, appeared to be integrating into the local schools attended by the island children.

Art therapy on Prvic

On-site work in Croatia was a three-week pilot project consisting of what was termed 'art sessions'. ATI were sent by UNHCR to the island of Prvic on the Dalmatian Coast. ATI's brief was to demonstrate to the head psychologist how short-term art therapy could be used at a refugee centre. They were informed that they would be working on 'a small island in a refugee centre with severely traumatised individuals' – mainly children.

The pilot art therapy project intended to involve all members of the centre in the art-making process. The psychologists had already attempted to provide talking groups but without success in sustaining them. They had also established a drama and dance group which proved more successful, although intermittent. ATI's intention was to offer art sessions as art therapists. As at Hrastnik, ATI aimed to offer facilitated art sessions, responding to the themes and images that emerged through the art-making process. The word 'theme' used in the following diary is used loosely to refer to either the emerging theme or the art material presented for that session. As at Hrastnik, a regular structure was attempted but was difficult to maintain due to the complex school timetable in place. It was however possible to offer art each day: ATI intended to respond to the context and the structures already in place.

In contrast to Hrastnik, Prvic centre was defined as a temporary situation. It was also newly established and the refugees had only lived at the centre for five months maximum (in one case, one week). Because refugees at Hrastnik had already lived there for up to two years, they had already become familiar with the routine of refugee life and had established a community of some sort at Hrastnik centre. Those arriving at Prvic were coming from a variety of situations – either recently arriving from Bosnia directly or from other refugee centres or local towns. Therefore each person was caught in their own story and came with different needs and burdens. Because there were only 24 refugees, ATI was able to become familiar with the story of each individual in the centre (Appendix 3). ATI was also able to record in the diary each person's use of the art sessions.

All psychological support offered at the centre had to be short-term and focused due to its transitional nature. This pilot art therapy project was clearly defined in a three week time-frame with no future visits intended. The continuing presence of the psychologist and social worker made possible follow-up psychological support where necessary.

ATI used only local art materials, available in Sibenik. Meetings of groups took place in the dining room. This provided ATI with a challenge to create a place conducive to immersion in art-making in a communal living space. There were up to four art sessions each day. The groups were divided according to age: small children, school-age children, adolescents and adults.

Individuals were encouraged to explore their own themes and to experiment with the art materials. The art sessions were structured in what ATI called an 'open structure'. In this structure ATI offered containing elements through the different art materials they presented on each day (for example, the size of paper, shape of paper) and allowed or facilitated whatever image manifested itself. Paintings and drawings ranged from very large to postcard-sized.

Children responded to the simple availability of the art materials. In the early sessions it was not unusual for one child to produce a dozen paintings in the space of an hour. In response to this ATI introduced small pieces of paper – postcard size – and this appeared to provide a focus for both the individual and the artwork: the images changed, becoming more detailed and less muddy. Adults and adolescents began in organised sessions but became a self-motivated group of individuals. They painted or drew whenever they had time or inclination. ATI's contact with them was therefore largely informal as they would come requesting art materials and gather in the dining room or take them to their room and return with the paintings at a later stage.

The following is a diary of day-to-day art sessions and general observations made over the three-week period.*

The inclusion of the diary provides details which would be lost in any other form. All refugees' names have been changed for the purposes of confidentiality.

- Morning sessions: 10.00 am–12.00 pm
- Afternoon sessions 1.00 pm–3.00 pm/4.00 pm
- Late afternoon sessions: 4.00 pm–6.00 pm
- Evening sessions: 5.00 pm–7.00 pm

Session times were governed by changing ferry timetables which alternated weekly.

Day One
Afternoon: Arrival on the island. Orientation, observation and assessment. Meeting with volunteers, refugees and the centre's psychologist, Natasa, and social worker, Mari. On this day ATI became familiar with the environment and tried to understand the daily structures and routines.

- *Orientation and observation:* Lethargy and lack of structure. General feedback from workers was that it would be impossible to motivate the refugees. Awareness of how necessary it was to identify the lethargy in order not to be drawn into it.

Day Two
Morning: Meeting with psychologist and social worker – briefing on the history of the refugee centre and individual case histories, meeting with the director and his assistant, agreement upon ATI's mandate: aims, objectives, time span, and practical requirements.

Afternoon: Converted an unused bedroom into an art therapy room.

Evening: Informal art group with small children (2–8-year-olds) in newly prepared art room. Mario, Mari, Blazenka, Ljuba, Hukmeta, Refija. Children came readily to

*See Appendix 3 for more details, observations and information on each individual.

explore art room, art materials and boundaries of the art groups in this new setting.
Theme: introductions.
Summary: The children seemed to want to introduce themselves to Bobby and Debra through their images.

- *Orientation and observation:* Continued sense of lethargy and lack of direction.

Day Three
Morning: Visit to elderly refugee centre at Vodice.*

Afternoon: Children's art group. Mario, Hikmeta, Mari, Mirela, Blazenka, Refija. Continuation from previous day. *Theme:* introductions.
Significant interactions: The children used quantities of material, pouring paint to make picture after picture.
Summary: The children seemed to be excited by the mere provision of the art materials.

Evening: Informal socialising with volunteers and refugees.

- *Orientation and observation:* Lethargy felt less pervasive.

Day Four
Morning: Boat to Sibenik to buy art materials.

Afternoon: Teenage and adult art group. Theme: Introduction to art and art processes through Polaroids and drawing/painting. Each person invited to take one Polaroid photograph of any detail visible from within the room, followed by a drawing or painting of a section or the whole image. Fourteen participants. Zlatka, Mina (with baby, Ivan), Stephan (volunteer), Ermin, Emir, Azra, Adisa, Natasa, Mari, Bobby, Debra, Cook, Elvis, Gorana.
Aim: A 'non-threatening' introduction to using art.
General atmosphere: Industriousness and involvement, with long periods of quiet, concentrated art-making. Initial encouragement of participation necessary, and made through individual invitations. Also, coffee and music.
Significant interactions:
- Zlatka worked with quiet concentration for an extended period.
- Ermin arrived late, said he didn't want to paint but soon had taken a Polaroid which he then abandoned. Instead he made three drawings: cartoon-like caricatures; a picture of a clown which he coloured in; a cat which he traced.
- Emir came late, was at first ambivalent and then took a Polaroid of the art cupboard and produced a striking, brightly coloured image. He seemed proud of it.
- Azra was apprehensive and yet painted two landscape images.
- Elvis took a Polaroid and remained on the outside of the group, being present but not drawing.
- Gorana produced a careful image of her hand with red manicured nails, taken from a polaroid and her traced hand. (Later it became apparent that this picture visually represented her preoccupation with her physical appearance – and her hands in particular. Although she was often present in future art groups, this was her only complete image.)

*See 'Refugee centres in Croatia'.

Summary: Astonished by the level of involvement at this early stage and in view of expectations resulting from earlier feedback.

• *Orientation and observation:* Sense of lethargy not present this afternoon. Atmosphere generally industrious and involved: a sense of interest.

Day Five
Morning: Organised walk around the island.

Afternoon: The director ordered the dismantling of the art room and directed that the art groups be held in the main dining area. Following this, reactions were varied: some rebelled against this decision while most of the adolescents seemed to gain energy and enjoyment in 'pulling down' the created space.

Evening: Open art group for all ages. Attended by most of the refugees including mothers, adolescents, and children (Fig. 12). *Theme:* open.
Significant interactions: A stream of images was produced in this session, with individuals asking for more and more paper. Refija (mother of Hikmeta) participated by 'correcting' Hikmeta's work. Elma (mother of Mari, Mario, Blazenka and Mirela) made her first and last image, as did Dejan who made a football drawing as his first communication and introduction to the art sessions. Daniel (volunteer) made a stylised painting of the island.
Summary: The quantity of images expressed in one session was overwhelming. There was a sense that there was no end to these images. ATI considered that this perhaps represented 'spilling' of emotion and a very real need for the refugees to express themselves and their quantities of feeling.

• *Orientation and observation:* Charged atmosphere, with what appeared to be anger simmering beneath the surface and a frustration which was palpable. This continued until the following evening when there was an eruption of 'rebellious', high-spirited behaviour and seemed to result from a negative interaction between the director and the refugees. The director had visited at lunch and delivered a speech with a list of apparently unsubstantiated grievances supported by a series of new rules. This was met with silence and expressionless faces of the majority of the adolescents and adults. (Included in the new rules was the immediate dismantling of the newly prepared art room.)

Day Six
Morning: Art group with children. Mario, Hikmeta, Mari, Mirela, Blazenka, Mehmed, Ermin, Zarina. All the children joined in at different times. Emir was also present and, as an older member, his presence seemed to ground the group. Theme: Open. The *island* became the dominant theme of this group (and many groups to come). About thirty-five paintings made. Several of the children were inspired by Daniel's island image, and began to copy and then gradually develop it in their own way.
Significant interactions: Refija drew over Hikmeta's image with a 'correction'. Hikmeta was also the target for Ermin's teasing, and this was becoming a frequent dynamic between Hikmeta and various other children.
Summary: The children's need to use up so much paper and materials seemed to be becoming a routine as well as to symbolise their enormous and unmet emotional needs. Adolescents joined in on their own motivation.

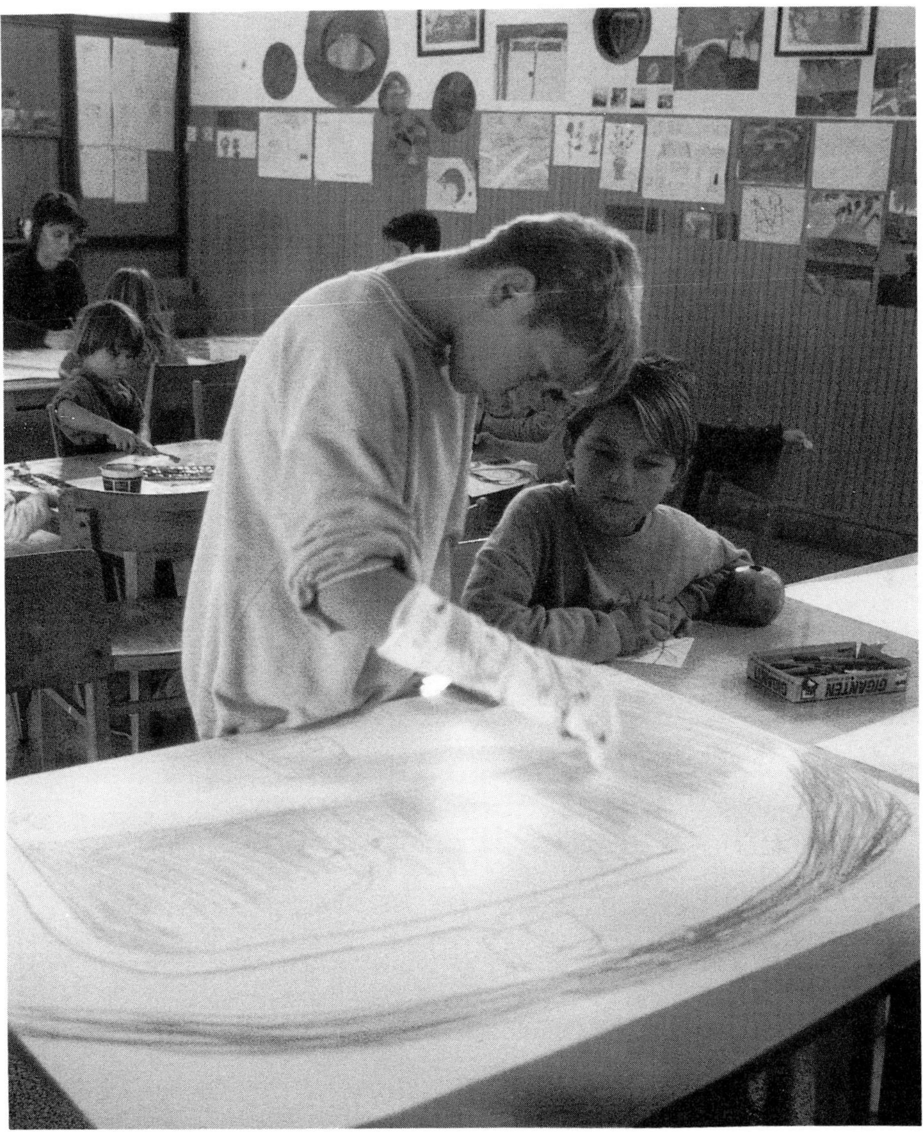

Figure 12. Group art session, for all ages, in the communal dining area, Prvic refugee centre

Afternoon: Painting with children and adults. *Theme:* Mandalas: choice of small and large circles. Emir, Stephan, Azra, Ljuba, Selver, Refija and Cook's daughter. A quiet group with changing energy levels.

Significant interactions: Emir spent the whole day painting, beginning after breakfast and stopping only for lunch. He painted landscapes from his imagination and then from postcards: sensitive use of paint. Refija made her first painting – carefully painted flowers in a vase. When it was suggested that she might think about placing the painting on the wall (selecting an image and taping it to the wall had become a way of ending each group) she looked both a little embarrassed and pleased, and said – through an interpreter – that it was like a seven-year-old's drawing, and would be a bad influence on Hikmeta's development. Mario and Mari were running in and out of the dining room, and becoming disruptive and very demanding. The only thing that appeared to calm them was the physical touch of a massage to face and brow.

Summary: Emir's continuing and enthusiastic involvement with the art-making was noteworthy in that it was inconsistent with his truancy and reported lack of interest and inability to concentrate at school. It was apparent that physical touch – although always needing to be used with awareness and care – played an important role in holding and containing some of the young children and seemed to be the only way of doing so at this stage.

Evening: The director had left the centre this evening after staying for two days during which the atmosphere had been subdued and controlled. On the director's departure, the dining room tables were strewn with empty wine bottles, which was notable in the light of the new rule: no alcohol allowed on the premises. (Bobby and Debra later discovered that this was an act of defiance with empty bottles taken from the dustbins.) The tension was also demonstrated by incidents witnessed: there was an exceptional quiet throughout the building; Refija, normally withdrawn, was seen running through the centre in pursuit of Hikmeta and hitting her; Elvis, a boy of sixteen, appeared to take on the role of 'carer' in the centre. (His room was often the venue for night gatherings, a cosier space in which he usually provided music and coffee.) On this evening, Elvis had moved into the corridor and was providing vitamins and bandages to anyone that passed.

• *Orientation and observation:* The day began calmly, developed into an atmosphere of defiance and ended with a tension that was all-pervasive and with a source that was hard to identify.

Day Seven

Morning: Meeting with Natasa and Mari to discuss observations and general concerns. It was discovered that these visits from the director were fortnightly, but that this meeting and atmosphere was the most concerning to date. In addition, Natasa and Mari had been reproached for the lack of control in the centre. They said that they feared the disintegration of the structure: that refugees would begin to leave. The rest of the meeting involved listening to their anger, fears and concerns in this work.

Afternoon: Group with small children. *Theme:* Mandala. Mirela, Mihana, Blazenka, Mehmed, Zarina, Hikmeta, nurse (Ana), Mari. This group was calm and contained.

- *Orientation and observation:* 'Hugo': south wind brought by the sea, warm and carrying with it a dense air pressure; strong winds; unusually rough sea; heavy grey skies; several complaints of oppressive headaches and depressive feelings.

Day Eight
Morning: Boat to Sibenik to buy art materials, followed by informal painting group with younger children on the terrace. Mirela, Hikmeta, Mehmed, Mihana, Zarina, Mari, Mario. Nurse joined in. *Theme:* painting, and introduction of Plasticine.

Afternoon: Children's group. *Theme:* Clay. Mirela, Hikmeta, Mehmed, Mihana, Zarina, Mari, Mario. Each individual was given a piece of clay and a board. The work began with a tentative exploration, in which children attempted to make recognisable objects.
Significant interactions: Mari introduced water, but left before she became more involved. The rest of the group adopted this new material and the water allowed them to use the clay in a more primary way – splashing and playing with the clay as an end in itself.
Summary: This was the first session which seemed to develop its own pace, and in which the children were working within this therapeutic structure as a group. The fact that Mari withdrew before getting more deeply involved was noted as consistent with her previous behaviour.

Evening: Adolescents independently collected paper and art materials to take back to their rooms, or dining area. (Most of them brought their paintings back to show Bobby and Debra at a later stage.)
Significant interactions: Adisa worked on a painting for an hour, then tore it up saying 'I hate it; it looks like a child's drawing. Before the war it was not like this.'

- *Orientation and observation:* The storm had subsided and the day was generally calmer and passed without event.

Day Nine
Morning: Meeting with Natasa and Mari. Discussion of their work and concerns, including dynamics, problems, possible solutions, dreams, etc., and refugee family groups and histories. An issue of importance raised was their lack of, and need for, supervision.

Morning: Small children's groups. Natasa and Mari were present. Mirela, Refija, Mihana, Mehmed. *Theme:* Postcard drawing. Outside in the sun, it was calm and quiet.

Afternoon: Mixed group – all ages. *Theme:* Postcards. Azra, Mina and Ivan, Hikmeta, Ljuba, Mirela, Mario, Mari.
Significant interactions: Mari was able to stay with the group on this occasion and produced finished work. Azra chose to paint her own interpretation of two postcards and was absorbed in the process.
Summary: The small pieces of paper appeared to act for Mari as a containing element and allowed her to focus in more detail on her images. (This development remained and Mari chose this sized paper in most of the subsequent sessions.)

Evening: Organised walk up the hill above the centre with adolescents and adults.
* *Orientation and observation:* another calm day.

Day Ten
Morning: Painting group with small children. *Theme:* Painting of found-wood pieces. Introduction of acrylic paints.
Afternoon: Painting with older children. *Theme:* Open.
Significant interactions: Disparate group which took place on the patio, with fighting amongst the children. Hikmeta was visibly upset and painted a girl with a 'happy' face and red dots covering her body.

Afternoon: Art group outside with older children and adolescents. *Theme:* Art walk, photographs using throwaway camera. The intention was for each person to take photographs of their environment. Initially the walk revolved around the camera, starting as exciting and soon leading to fights and difficulties in sharing. The energy was disparate and hard to contain. The walk continued for a while along the rocks. On their return, Mari and Mario insisted on climbing upon a tiny chapel above the rocks, from which Mario leapt and cut his knee. This was followed by a more subdued return to the centre. Later, Mirela made a line drawing which seemed to depict herself and her brother with Mario limping and Mirela following in the same stance.

Evening: Adolescents continued painting informally.

* *Orientation and observation:* On beginning the groups on this day the atmosphere was a little unsettled, and it was difficult to create a structure. In the morning the nurse bandaged the little children's hands and fingers as a game. By the evening, Ermin had a bandage on his hand and fingers set in plaster; Mario's knee was bandaged; and Dejan's arm was bandaged after he had cycled off the pier into the sea. Although the bandages may have appeared coincidental, their prevalence was striking.

Day Eleven
Morning: Meeting with Natasa to review and discuss final week's programme.

Morning: Group with small children. *Theme:* Plasticine. Mirela, Mehmed, Blazenka, Mihana. The group took place outside, sheltered from the wind. There was laughter and more energy, and the group felt more cohesive.

Afternoon: Older children's group inside. *Theme:* Individual collage leading to group painting. Mirela, Zarina, Mari, Mario, Hikmeta, Mehmed. This group began with much fighting, but towards the end the group came together and resulted in some harmonious and productive work.
Significant interactions: For the first time the children shared paints and seemed actively aware of one another's work – borrowing shapes and colours from each other. As a result, a large sheet of paper was introduced and a communal group piece suggested. What became clear was that most of the children were not yet ready to work as a group and were unable to share the paper and therefore created their own space within it. They also returned to their individual pieces. Zarina and Mari worked well together however – starting with drawing and moving on to a collage, which they managed to share. They appeared to calm and ground each other.

- *Orientation and observation:* 'Hugo' storm – winds and rain. Various individuals complained of headaches. It appeared impossible to underestimate the influence of the weather on this island. The elements were acknowledged by the villagers as influential in their day-to-day physical existence and their moods.

Day Twelve (Sunday)
Morning and afternoon: 10.00 am–5.00 pm. Large group – all ages, grouped at different tables with different materials. *Theme:* For children: free drawing and painting on small paper and at a separate table. For adolescents and adults: large sheets of paper and acrylics, and optional theme of Prvic Island. There was a brief break for lunch, by which time the dining room was a hive of activity.
12.30 pm–4.30 pm Bobby and Debra attended a meeting in Sibenik with ARC. The group continued with its own momentum through the afternoon.
Significant interactions: Mari was influenced by Ljuba's concentration, and moved from paint to crayon. Hikmeta began painting with the group of children until her mother joined her in order to coach her in drawing a house and a tree. The other children left the table, leaving mother and daughter alone. Azra concentrated on a large painting for several hours – surprising herself by its strength and cohesion, and depicting the island with houses and roads. The theme of roads and paths, introduced by Emir in one of the first sessions, was adopted by Azra and others. Elvis painted a flower and a butterfly on a large sheet. He also allowed another member of the group to make a pencil portrait of Elvis on this same sheet, working side by side.
Summary: It was observed that in the images of houses and roads, the roads were almost invariably left unpainted with paths leading off them. Azra had begun a large drawing and planned to continue it the next day (Kalmanowitz and Lloyd, 1997, unpublished).

- *Orientation and observation:* After lunch, due to a pre-arranged meeting with ARC in Sibenik, the group continued in ATI's absence, with Emir accepting responsibility for the materials. It was not possible to change the meeting due to the lack of access to a telephone. Leaving the group was an uncomfortable necessity. However, it was useful in that it gave the opportunity for the group to function independently and was particularly important in view of ATI's imminent departure from the island. It was reported that the group stayed together, and had worked well and found its own momentum; the materials had been cared for and the paintings were taped to the wall.

Day Thirteen
Morning: Informal adolescent group on patio. *Theme:* Plasticine.

Afternoon: Children and adolescents in two groups. *Theme:* Chalk drawing on patio floor outside. The children drew as a group in their marked-out area. The adolescents however, were unable and/or unwilling to work as a group but used the chalk separately this day and on subsequent days not only on the allocated area but in the entire outside environment (including drawing on the pier outside the centre's fence, on paved areas inside the grounds and on the table tennis table).

Afternoon: Adolescent art group. *Theme:* Continuation of paintings on large paper.
Significant interactions: Azra continued her careful pencil drawing of a church. Mario joined in and appeared preoccupied: he scribbled on small pieces of paper with great force, later slicing through these images making them into loosely held shreds.
Summary: Mario's previous images were consistent with his behaviour of the

previous day: it was discovered that the dead cat found outside the kitchen had been strangled by Mario. (This was apparently not the first time.)

Evening: Beginning of portrait photographs taken by ATI. Formal individual and family photographic portraits in response to requests.

• *Orientation and observation:* Art materials were available all day. There was an undercurrent of lethargy which again turned into a full day and became easier as it advanced. This day began slowly with the adolescents playing with the plasticine outside in the sun.

Day Fourteen
Morning: Walk with children to their school on the island and to the boat for Sibenik. No art groups.

Afternoon: Boat to Obanjan – island for refugees and displaced people.* Accompanied by Elvis (former resident on Obanjan, Elvis wanted to visit his friends and this was a rare opportunity for this to take place as it was difficult to gain access to the island). Meeting with psychologists and refugees.

Day Fifteen
Morning: Return to Prvic. 'Day of the Dead' – This day was a national holiday and therefore no school. Art materials were made available for general use but not in a formal group structure. Beginning of recording process of images in slide form (with consent of individuals).

Afternoon: Art group, all ages. No theme. Mario, Blazenka, Mari, Hikmeta, Refija, Azra.

Day Sixteen
Morning and afternoon: Slide taking for documentation of images – with consent of individuals.
Significant interactions: Supper: Refija slapped Hikmeta across the face and Hikmeta stared back blank-faced. This display of aggression was alarming in that it was made so public. Zlatka immediately came to Hikmeta's defence, emotively expressed her anger at this unprovoked act and left the dining area. This lead to an informal discussion, between the group of those present, on the theme of mothering, caring, mother and child relationships and the importance of physical touch. (The following day, Zlatka and Refija continued with the discussion.)

Day Seventeen
This was the final day.
Morning: Boat to Sibenik to buy film and materials. Completion of slide documentation.

Afternoon: Closing group, with children. Mario, Hikmeta, Blazenka, Mari, Mirela, Zarina, Refija. High energy level in this session and a palpable sense of this being the last painting group in this format with ATI. *Theme:* Open. Acrylic painting, drawing and painting of clay pieces.
Significant interactions: As in the very first sessions the children used an excessive amount of materials – pouring, dripping and layering the paint until the paper

*See 'Refugee Centres in Croatia'

became saturated and could not hold it. The paint took hours to dry and was still wet at supper time.
Summary: The afternoon was one of intense involvement and seemed a return to the layering and using up of paint and paper as at the beginning of the three weeks.

Evening: Farewell party. Each person was handed a folder of their art work and invited to select a piece to be taken back to London by ATI. There was astonishment amongst the refugees that the folders had been carefully kept and individuals reviewed their work over the last three weeks, some surprising themselves as to work they had produced, while others discussed the experience of making art on a daily basis. The party continued with informal discussions of the pictures covering the walls, and there was a mixture of pride and indifference towards the images. This was followed by food, music and dancing.

• *Orientation and observation:* The mood of the party was festive with energetic dancing and singing which carried on into the night. The ambivalent response to the folders and art work on the walls was noted after the intense and focused involvement during the art-making.

Conclusion

Prvic refugee centre was a place of transition. Refugees lived there with the intention of moving on: they seemed, to a greater or lesser extent, to be camping in their rooms and there was a sense of endless waiting, of lethargy and aimlessness. Unlike Hrastnik where there appeared to be an acceptance of the situation with the women spending most of their time cleaning and maintaining their immediate environment, at Prvic the communal spaces were mostly uncared for. (Any cleaning that was carried out in the communal areas was done so by a Croatian woman, employed to clean the building.) At Hrastnik there was a sense of a 'community', in which the roles the women adopted presented not only clean barracks but represented an attempt to create a functioning home. Prvic, by contrast, had a sense of a dysfunctional home with no one taking on the role of parent.

The reaction to the folders (see 'Day Seventeen') is one example of the ambivalence that pervaded the atmosphere of the centre. Beyond a general surprise that the folders had been carefully kept, most of the folders were still on the tables the following morning. Over the three weeks, the art-making had been intense and focused, with individuals requesting art materials between sessions and showing a sense of interest and pride. This was in contrast to the general atmosphere in which spare time was used aimlessly. Throughout the three weeks there had been a sense of a bottomless pit in the lives of this group of people and an expectation that ATI could and should fill it. A tangible expression of this was the constant demand for more art materials, coffee, cigarettes, claiming of personal possessions. The art sessions attempted to provide a space in which individuals could begin to discover, or rediscover, their internal resource and a language of expression upon which they could build.

All 23 individuals made art at one time or another and no one way was typical. A more detailed account of four individuals living at the centre at this time and their use of the art sessions shows four personal responses to the art, demonstrating very different uses and the subtlety of intervention that three weeks of art sessions offered.

Emir (16 years old) arrived from a village in Bosnia near Zenica with his two siblings just before the war began. They arrived at Prvic after a period in another camp in Croatia. The three are the youngest of a family of ten, the rest of whom remained with their parents in Bosnia. One of the points ATI were told about Emir was that he was one of the more disruptive members of his class and frequently played truant from school. The first art session Emir arrived late and with an ambivalence. From then on he was an enthusiastic member of the art sessions and painted almost daily, and at the weekend sometimes the whole day, joining any group or initiating his art-making – requesting art materials. One of his first images was that of a village, with roads and paths leading off them. This seemed to hold significance for the group as when Emir pinned it the wall similar images on the same theme painted or drawn by different people followed over the subsequent days. Towards the end of ATI's stay, Emir expressed that he had seldom painted before and requested a set of paints for his personal use after ATI had left.

Mirela (4 years old) was born in Sarajevo and stayed at the centre with her mother (Elma) and three siblings. As a result of the actions of her father, the family was threatened with blood revenge focusing on her brother. Due to this and in conjunction with the war Elma had to flee Sarajevo with her family. This family had been refugees for two years. During the three weeks, Mirela participated in all of the art groups and illustrated an acute ability to absorb and learn. On speaking to Elma ATI learned that Mirela had had very little opportunity in the past two years to paint or draw or participate in any such activity. Indeed, what ATI witnessed was that the very young children ran around the island most of the day entertaining themselves. Mirela seemed to be stimulated by the art-making, she painted and drew and on one occasion seemed to discover, to her surprise, that she had created green. On another occasion after a long period of drawing she began to shout excitedly 'kuca , kuca' ('house' in Serbo-Croat); it appeared that this was a realisation that she could name what she had drawn. It was also the first representation ATI had seen of a house in her drawings. She then filled a number of pages with houses.

Elvis (17 years old), was born in Bosnia, is the youngest of eleven brothers and sisters and the only member of his family living at Prvic Refugee Centre. The information surrounding Elvis and his family history is incomplete and confused. It is understood that Elvis lived in Croatia for several years before the war began, spending time in a school for children with 'mental disturbance' with one of his sisters, and in a psychiatric unit in Zagreb. He then was moved to Obanjan refugee centre for a year before arriving on Prvic. Since then, Elvis had displayed self-abusive behaviour, had threatened another resident and hit out at some of the small children. Although Elvis was greatly liked in the centre he was also feared for his unpredictable behaviour. He was the only individual in the centre with his own bedroom and he would often disappear from the life of the centre for hours or days; staying up all night and sleeping all day, or locking himself in his room, ignoring all knocks and calls. Despite this, Elvis seemed to have an acute sensitivity towards both his immediate environment and the indivduals in it and would respond with both practical and creative solutions. On the night before the storm, (art therapy on Prvic: day six) for example, when the atmosphere in the centre was particularly tense and unsettled, Elvis distributed bandages and vitamin C tablets from his self-assembled first aid kit. This seemed to arise from a desire to care for those around him and a need to make sense of his own situation. He joined the art sessions when he became familiar with ATI's way of working. This pleasantly surprised everybody as Elvis generally did not join organised activities. His first painting was on a large sheet of paper, depicting a bold and bright flower and butterfly. He allowed another member of the group to make a pencil portrait of himself on this same sheet, working side by side. It was not so much the content of the images as the fact that he was able to be part of the group art-making that seemed notable.

Zlatka (33 years old) is a nurse and was originally from Tusla. Zlatka's husband, parents and parents in-law all remained in Bosnia. Zlatka is a Muslim and the family lived in a Serb area. Her husband is a Bosnian Serb and as a soldier was unable to leave. Zlatka and her two children left her husband and Tusla in April 1992 and had been refugees in Croatia for less than a year. What characterised Zlatka was her determination to look ahead and to provide her children with a future. She was in the process of applying for refugee status in Switzerland. She expressed on more than one occasion that there was no place for regrets. This was in spite of the fact that she had both physical and emotional problems of her own which were exacerbated by alcohol. Zlatka spent much of her spare time in the sewing room designing and making clothes which provided her with a small income. Her involvement in art-making was with the same determination with which she approached her life. When she found the energy she painted large and said that she felt that it helped her pass time constructively and sometimes helped with her strong emotions.

Themes
In the above context, ATI would like to highlight two main themes that recurred as they emerged from the group over the three- week period: the images of islands and roads arose in different individual's paintings either simultaneously in the same session or in subsequent sessions so that eventually there were collections of roads and islands covering the walls of the dining room. As it was not ATI's intention at this stage to discuss the images with each person or the group unless this was initiated by the individual, it is difficult to know what the themes represented for the artist at the time of making. Images hold multiple meanings and it is therefore only possible to propose suggestions about the images as connected to each individual in the particular context. It is acknowledged that the images discussed are symbolic, metaphoric and rich in meaning.

Emir was the first to introduce the theme of roads, which, as has already been mentioned, was to become a recurring theme in the group (Figs. 13–15, Pl. 4). 'Roads have been universally significant since their development some 5000 years ago. Their mythic and metaphoric meaning has permeated the language, art, poetry and music of virtually all cultures' (Hanes, 1995, p. 19). Most of the roads appearing in the art-work of the group cross the page and lead off it; there is usually a house or series of houses lining the road, and often a crossroad or tributary path leading from the main road. On reflecting on the images of roads made in this context, there is a clear sense that this was an image that held meaning, perhaps representing the past, present and future: maps of villages in Bosnia, homes with roads leading nowhere and cross-roads.

The island first emerged in the image of a volunteer who painted a silhouetted piece of land in the middle of the sea, with a palm tree and orange sunset. This theme was taken up by many of the children first and then adopted by the adolescents and adults later. Some of the children painted the island repeatedly over a period of days. The refugees were living on an island and the images could therefore represent the 'here and now'. *An Illustrated Encyclopaedia of Traditional Symbols* describes an island:

'Ambivalent as a place of isolation and loneliness but also a place of safety and refuge from the sea of chaos' (Cooper, 1978 p. 88).

It is integral in an art therapy group for common themes to emerge in the art-work of individuals. Although the images may appear to be copied one from the other, it is understood that they emerge spontaneously and unconsciously with one individual responding to the image of another and interpreting it for his / her own use. The theme resonates on different levels at various times for different individuals and this experience often evokes new material, new insights. What members have in common, collectively and inherently, emerges in the images made by the individuals in the group and therefore the unconscious can be seen as providing the theme of the group. The roads and the islands emerged as the two most visible themes amongst the group, although each individual of course expressed idiosyncratic themes in his/her own art work.

These thoughts are intended to offer a sympathetic understanding so as to expand, rather than limit, options.

Art-making managed to cross language barriers, it demanded active participation of individuals, helping to combat apathy and boredom. The art-making seemed to help Emir, for example, to gain in self-esteem; for Refija the art-making appeared to offer the beginning of reflection; for others, such as Mario and Mari, art sessions seemed to be cathartic, providing a contained space in which to express emotions (see Diary above and Appendix 3). Above all, however, the art sessions seemed to provide a forum, a structure in which different groups gathered, socialised and communicated, which in this context seemed of great value.

In addition to the above, ATI concluded from the art therapy pilot project that the psychologist and social worker at Prvic refugee centre (they also provided psychological support to the elderly refugee centre at Vodice) needed support and regular supervision to enable them to continue with their work and replenish their energies. They were exhausted and this was their first job for which they were receiving no professional back-up. This corresponded with ATI's findings from Sarajevo, Mostar and Zagreb in which local carers and professionals themselves needed support, were often 'burnt-out' and in need of supervision and training (see footnote, p. 76). ATI was able to recommend to Social Services, UNHCR, Split that the psychologist and social worker urgently need regular clinical supervision in order to continue offering useful psychological support to the refugees.

In conclusion, ATI found on Prvic an extreme situation in which art played an important role as a subtle intervention. As art therapists, the role was to responsibly facilitate expression and to follow the lead of each individual rather than impose a structure. However, as already stated, a pervading sense of emptiness that asked to be filled was present throughout the three weeks. It was clear that in this context the art sessions could not and should not attempt to fill this, despite the constant discomfort ATI experienced of not being good enough or offering enough. The art sessions attempted to provide a space in which a seed could be planted which would have a life after the three-week period, and upon which individuals could build.

Update 1996

Hrastnik refugee centre

The following update was received from the Bosnian Support Group in September 1996: since the Dayton Peace agreement in December 1995, news from Bosnia has begun to filter through to Hrastnik: news of relatives' injuries and deaths, of homes damaged or destroyed or now in areas designated 'Serb'. Most of the refugees are anxious, depressed and fearful for the future. Many do not believe the peace will hold. The Slovenian government has now given permission for the camp to remain open for at least 15 more months, until December 1997. Some refugees are choosing to stay in Slovenia when this is possible, or to go to Croatia rather than return home. Those returning to Bosnia are making their way back individually. The resident volunteer, Bernard, has personally driven refugees to Kljuc, to villages near Serb-occupied Brcko, to Kamengrad, Bosanski Petrovac, to Tuzla, Teocak and Sanski Most. Refugees whose homes are in Serb-held Bosnia are only allowed to visit the Federation if looking for a place to live.

Conditions in Hrastnik refugee centre itself have deteriorated: the food quality is worse, 50 new refugees have arrived from Sevnica, a camp which has recently closed, bringing temporary chaos and discomfort to Hrastnik. Most of these refugees come from the Serb-occupied territory of Doboj; many are sick. There is still no psychological support at Hrastnik, although the hut built in 1994 is used now for a nursery school, English classes and other camp activities. Children still continue to play with 'boundless energy'. The mood of the refugees – confused, resigned, but often coloured with humour – has largely turned to frustration as a result of all the increased uncertainties.

The Bosnian Support Group intends to continue to support Hrastnik refugees over the next 15-month period, particularly those with no home to return to, giving money according to need to all families returning, to enable them to re-start their lives in Bosnia or Croatia.

Prvic refugee centre

The following update was received in a recent communication through Social Services UNHCR in Split, Croatia in September 1996 via the UNHCR office in London: the centre is still running and there are now between 38 and 40 children, adolescents and mothers living in Prvic refugee centre. The criteria for the camp remains for 'traumatised children and single mothers'. It is believed the same level of psychological support is still being offered.

Art therapy in the former Yugoslavia

The following update was received in May 1996 from aid organisations working in the former Yugoslavia, through letters, printed information, telephone conversations and computer-search print-outs. These were followed up by ATI with questionnaires.

ATI contacted the organisations in order to understand whether they are aware of any art or art therapy projects taking place in the former Yugoslavia at this time. Out of the ten organisations contacted, only UNICEF returned the questionnaire (Appendix 4).

The following questions were asked in the questionnaire, in relation to art therapy in the former Yugoslavia:

- Do you know of any art projects that exist or have existed?
- Do you know of any art therapy projects that exist or have existed?
- Did you come across any informal art-making taking place?
- Have you come across any written documentation on art or art therapy in this context?
- How do you understand art therapy?
- Any other information or questions?

The summary below sets out the most recent findings:

- The Serious Road Trip carried out a programme called True Colours in Central Bosnia between October 1995 and January 1996, run by artists and musicians. The work involved mural painting with children in institutions and value was placed on both the process and product. Most of the images were of houses or fantasy and only one image depicted the war directly. The group referred to a child psychologist carrying out art projects and a freelance British art therapist and music therapist working in Zenica. The Serious Road Trip said they had come across what was termed 'art therapy' in Bosnia which involved people being asked to paint their war experience.

- Medact continues to send child psychotherapists, psychiatrists and other medically trained practitioners to work with teachers and social workers in the former Yugoslavia. Some have brought back children's drawings which they found of interest. Medact was very interested to hear of ATI's work and suggested they devise a questionnaire.

- Scottish European Aid offered art therapy projects in Romania, which were understood to be of great value but has no such projects in the former Yugoslavia.

- Marie Stopes International is offering art as a hobby which is passed on to other members of the women's groups which the organisation offers. They suggested that art therapy would fall under their occupational and educational work.

- Médecins sans Frontières offers no art or art therapy projects in the former Yugoslavia although they do have a successful art therapy programme in Rwanda.

- Action Aid is researching conflict and post-conflict situations with a community-based approach. They were very interested to receive ATI's report and to see whether it would fit into their education programmes.

- UNICEF offers the Step-by-Step to Recovery programme in which art workshops held in libraries throughout Croatia have become a focal point for children traumatised by war (Appendix 2).

- Oxfam conducted a computer-search into their programmes in the former Yugoslavia for ATI. The following art and health-related projects were found:

1. *Kids workshop in Serbia.* October 1994: 4 to 5 day workshops aiming 'to provide refugee children with opportunities for fun, creative and therapeutic activities which will enhance their living situation and outlook for the future' using animators. 'Women make up about 80 per cent of the refugee population in Serbia. In the absence of fathers, mothers are left to provide for all needs of their children. Through this project, Oxfam will include women in the programme, providing support and encouragement by involving them in the activities for their children.' Monitoring of the project aimed to lead to insight into the psychological needs of refugee children living in collective accommodation, and to recommendations for continuing assistance and support to children in collective centres.

2. *Pozega Recreational and Rehabilitation Project in Serbia.* July 1994: 'The psychological scars of displacement, loss of livelihood, and separation from family and friends is often compounded by inactivity and little opportunity for engagement in constructive or therapeutic activities'. Professional input, primarily from mental health teams, will provide informal counselling support for refugees participating in group activities. These will be part of a larger psychological programme aiming to motivate and encourage refugees to become active and offer them opportunities for integration within their surroundings. Main aims were to include encouragement and facilitation of creative skills.

3. *Psycho-social support to child refugees in Serbia.* August 1995: Psycho-social workshops to support children and families through the implementation of play and art workshops for children in three refugee reception centres in Serbia.

4. *Refugee theatre group 'The Sun'.* September 1995: Serbia: following performances in 28 collective centres throughout the former Yugoslavia, the refugee theatre intended to organise an exhibition of refugee children's art works as part of its activities.

Literature review

There is little literature directly on the subject of 'art therapy and political conflict' per se. However, in the past ten years papers have been written on the following: art therapy and trauma, or PTSD, art therapy following disaster, art therapy in connection with holocaust survivors, art therapy with refugees, art therapy with combat veterans. In addition, articles on art therapy and abuse provide another context from which information, although not directly related, can offer important points for consideration in working in the context of violence (overt, covert, physical, sexual or emotional).

Art-related projects already exist in situations of political conflict (UNICEF, 1996; Smythe and Lewer, 1992; Sogoric, 1992; Medact, 1994; Gal, 1995; Modric, 1994. Documentation exists for projects in Serbia, Croatia and Bosnia, Angola, Rwanda, Romania and the Philippines (see 'Update 1996'). These range from writing and poetry projects to music, drama, performance art and mural painting. However, these should not be confused with the continuing therapeutic support created through the discipline of art therapy (Sanderson, 1995; Golub, 1984; Seligman, 1991; Gregorian *et al.*, 1996; Klingman, Koenigsfeld and Markman 1987). Although documentation exists on projects carried out by individual art therapists there has, to date, been little collation of this material. The bibliographies provided in this document attempt to address this shortcoming.

The different uses of language in describing people being 'treated' is usually related to the cultural context and psychological paradigm being used. The following review attempts to keep to the terms used in each paper: client, victim, survivor, patient, individual, person. Where the masculine form is used, this is to be taken to mean masculine or feminine.

When speaking of their work, therapists repeatedly make reference to the privilege felt in being involved in this work, that is, in another human being sharing his/her story of physical and spiritual struggle, excruciating pain, numerous losses and humiliating degradation: this is seen as a rare honour.

Mary Sanderson (1995), in her paper 'Art therapy with victims of torture: a new frontier', writes about art therapy as a form of healing, rather than treatment. She discusses and expands on seven benefits of art therapy for victims of torture: providing a non-directive approach; enabling the expression of suppressed emotion; permitting the punishment of the torturer through the image; enabling the recovery of one's life story; enabling the survivor to face the worst through the art-making; helping the survivor grieve. She describes the context, the Canadian Centre for Victims of Torture in Toronto, where she has worked for two years with victims of state torture who arrive from all corners of the world suffering from the emotional, psychological and spiritual effects of torture.

She writes that it is the emotional, psychological and spiritual aspects of torture that have the most devastating and long-lasting effects. The purpose of torture is to extract information or a confession or often intimidate the victim and other potential dissidents from further political activity:

> It is also to make the victim betray himself and others. By his screams and submissions he turns himself into a lower animal in his own eyes. He loses his sense of dignity. He is rendered sub-human . . . The people who come to our centre and are referred for art therapy have seen evil in its most sinister forms. Many of them believe that their torturers have succeeded in making them sub-human and that their spirit is dead. The role of the art therapist, through the miracle of art, is to help them believe that they can live again. (Sanderson, 1995, p. 1)

Ms Sanderson writes that portraying images is so basic to humankind that many victims of torture turn to art even in remote and unlikely places. She speaks of aboriginal children in the Guatemalan forest, children in refugee camps in places such as Bosnia and Honduras finding an outlet for their pent-up feelings through the art they produce (as was ATI's experience and findings again and again wherever they went in the former Yugoslavia – art fulfilling a natural role). She says that even without the aid of adequate art supplies or the assistance of a trained art therapist, these 'and many other victims around the world are discovering the healing power of art' (Sanderson, 1995, p. 2).

In her conclusion she says that the rate of rehabilitation is high, as many torture victims were leaders in their community with strong, well-developed egos. What they need is a caring therapist who will take time to listen, and help them rebuild their self-esteem and sort out what has happened. By choosing to examine their past through art therapy her clients are choosing life.

Deborah Golub (1984), in her article 'Symbolic expression in post-traumatic stress-disorder: vietnam combat veterans in art therapy', explores the way in which the art process and art product enabled Vietnam veterans to integrate their war experiences into their lives, even ten years after the event, during which time the delay had not necessarily erased the need to express traumatic memories. Golub talks about 'the creation and transformation of symbols' as offering 'veterans a new approach toward achieving self-integration and mastering the trauma.'

Ms Golub writes that 'the most profoundly healing aspect of art therapy came neither from men's interactions with material, nor from my presentation of techniques. Rather, it arose from the human relationship. This therapeutic alliance, in turn, depended on the establishment of trust' (Golub, 1985, p. 287). She also suggests that there are phases in post-trauma art and offers her impression that early combat drawings are similar to the explosive release of traumatic images noted among Cambodian refugee children immediately after their escape from the Pol Pot regime and subsequent Vietnamese invasion. 'In the case of veterans, "catastrophic drawings" did not appear for years or were discontinued after non-veteran viewers rejected early attempts. Although veterans locked away their images of witnessed horror for over a decade, the delay did not necessarily erase the need to express traumatic memories. Now, given the chance, these veterans may have been embodying their death imprints for the first time. As time went on in art therapy, veterans supplemented representations of specific past events with contemporary themes and abstract renderings.' 'Veterans who claimed that they had not cried since

Vietnam depicted more tears in their work. They allowed their images to weep until they, too, could cry' (Golub, 1985, pp. 290–1).

Zivya Seligman (1995) in her paper 'Trauma and drama: a lesson from the concentration camps', presents another point of interest in her differentiation between PTSD (Post-traumatic stress disorder) and LTS (Life-threatening situations) – that is, any event which threatens our lives, our health, the loss of someone precious, or something vital to our existence and integrity. In exploring the possible role the creative arts played in helping people cope she writes 'it appears that people intuitively turn to creative activity as a way of dealing with the LTS'. She quotes Victor Frankl, a psychologist who was imprisoned in Auschwitz and the author of *Man's Search for Meaning* (Frankl, 1959):

> The intensification of inner life helped the prisoner find refuge from the emptiness, desolation and spiritual poverty of his existence, by letting him escape into the past . . . As the inner life of the prisoner tended to become more intense, he also experienced the beauty of art and nature as never before (Frankl, 1959, pp. 58–9).

David Johnson (1987) in 'The role of the creative arts therapies in the diagnosis and treatment of psychological trauma', discusses why the creative arts therapies might be a treatment of choice and presents a thorough discussion of the nature, diagnosis, and treatment of psychological trauma. He writes about the role art therapy has to play in gaining access to traumatic images and memories:

> Due to the dissociation of memories of the traumatic experience and the resulting disruption of the patients' ability to translate feeling states into words (i.e. alexithymia) gaining access to traumatic events is exceedingly difficult. Nevertheless this difficulty may be due not only to these psychological defences, but also to the nature of the neurological processes responsible for the encoding of the event. One of the truly remarkable facts about traumatic memories is that when they erupt in flashbacks or nightmares they are often an exact replica of the event, down to every detail, as if they were photographed . . . Unlike other memories that vary slightly each time they are recalled, traumatic events are recalled exactly the same each time. (Johnson, 1987, p. 9)

Because the encoding of traumatic memories may be via a 'photographic' visual process, visual media may offer unique means of gaining access to these traumatic images and memories by which they may come to consciousness.

Rosemarie Howard (1990), in 'Art therapy as an isomorphic intervention in the treatment of a client with post-traumatic stress disorder' quotes Ochberg and Fojtik (1984) in defining victimisation:

> A physical assault or threat of assault, in which physical damage or violation occurs, accompanied by a sense on the part of the victim of reduction in dominance and concomitant resignation or rage or both.

Ms Howard goes on to say that the authors differentiated between acute and chronic victimisation. She says, 'acute victimisation' is a single episode, regardless of duration. The victim does not remain in the presence of the oppressor and so has the opportunity to heal physically and psychologically. In contrast, repetitive trauma over time characterises 'chronic victimisation'. For the vulnerable person in the climate of oppression, victimisation becomes a way of life.

Karen Callaghan (1993), in her article 'Movement psychotherapy with adult survivors of political torture and organised violence', refers to clients who, wherever they are, experience a state of Continuous Traumatic Stress Disorder (CTSD) (a term used by the Organisation for Appropriate Social Services in South Africa, 1987), rather than PTSD . To quote, 'in the countries of the original repression they face ongoing terror, in exile they face legal limbo, host country hostility, fear for family and friends left behind and distrust of other members of their country in exile (Callaghan, 1993, p. 412).

Ms Callaghan raises some important issues relevant to this context: she discusses *cross-cultural issues* and describes how, in many non-western societies the emphasis is placed on connections between body, mind and spirit in the community, rather than the individual. She discusses the non-verbal cultural differences and stresses that, in considering cultural 'differences', universal emotions must not be ignored. 'A balance must be struck between the cultural and the universal: cultural differences can be explored, identified and valued' (Callaghan, 1993, p. 415).

She also raises the issue of *interpreters*: if they are used, they become part of the verbal and non-verbal interaction that develops between client and workers. They are often able to facilitate a better understanding of cultural differences but their presence can complicate the dynamics of the therapeutic relationship.

Ms Callaghan stresses that the work must be *client-centred:* there must be a flexibility and a willingness to challenge western models of rehabilitation. It is the client who points the way and, if health professionals are prepared to be flexible and look afresh at their models, then they will have something to offer.

Klingman, Koenigsfeld and Markman (1987), in their article 'Art activity with children following disaster: a preventive-oriented crisis intervention modality' discuss *short-term and crisis-intervention work*. There are often large numbers of individuals in need of support and it is important to do what is possible within the light of limited resources. In the article, a 'preventive-oriented crisis intervention modality' presents art therapy as a form of crisis intervention: the model was put in place following a collision between a train and a bus leading a convoy of 4 buses on a year-end school outing. The bus was thrown 150 feet. There were 22 deaths and 15 children were injured. The children in the three buses following were eye-witnesses. In response, and as part of an outreach programme, a 'creativity room', in which a wide range of art materials was freely available, was set up for six days in the school and was facilitated by an artist. Children came for a day, 20 minutes, an hour. In total, 94 art works were collected and 40 children participated. The images were discussed, comparisons and major advantages of the use of art in such a context summarised.

The authors concluded that both community-oriented psychologists and art therapists should study this method as a 'preventive' tool for the following reasons:
• Lowering of defences
• Releasing tension

- Making an art object or series of objects provides tangibility and permanence, which can be shared with peers.
- Art materials are usually available in a school setting (or scrap materials found in any community). These can be considered for use by therapists regardless of their individual discipline and professional orientation.
- A larger group can be reached with no 'stigma' attached.
- Those children (or adults) participating need not be in need of clinical treatment nor do they need to give a case history.
- Art can be a socially acceptable medium for revealing reactions in the context of school activities. The art counsellor or person facilitating the art need not be viewed as a stigmatising health professional.
- Through this method, the individuals can be helped to alter their thoughts, feelings and behaviour that might otherwise tend towards the 'destructive' and 'pathological'.

In conclusion, only the articles which ATI has been able to find in art therapy journals directly relating to art therapy and political conflict over the past ten years have been reviewed. There is, however, clearly a broader literature on the subject, as has already been stated, which can contribute to insight and understanding. For a more comprehensive list of articles researched by ATI see the Bibliography.

Conclusion to the research

On 14 December 1995, the Dayton Peace Agreement was signed in Paris, guaranteeing independence of Bosnia and signed by the leaders of Bosnia, Croatia and Serbia. This agreement signalled the beginning of the end of the war in the former Yugoslavia. In March 1996, the Tavistock Clinic in London held a trauma seminar entitled: 'War in Croatia and Bosnia–Herzegovina – Psychological Aftermath'. The guest speaker was Dr Tanja Franciskovic, a psychiatrist, group psychotherapist and manager of the PTSD Department of Rijeka Psychiatric Clinic, Croatia. The focus of Dr Franciskovic's talk was on what she called the 'post-war phase' and detailed the impact of war trauma on the life of the individual, the community and the professional.

Individual	**Community**	**Professional**
Behavioural	Identity	Performance of job
Spiritual	Structure	Motivation
Cognitive	Social institutions	Interpersonal
Emotional	Surroundings	Behavioural
Physical		

The structure of each community, social institutions and immediate surroundings in the republics of Croatia and Bosnia–Herzegovina have changed with the war. As a result, both these countries have been required to re-establish structures and adapt to new circumstances.* Since the Dayton Peace Agreement in December 1995, there has been a general increase of patients at the PTSD department of Rijeka Psychiatric Clinic. Dr Franciskovic explained this increase as directly relating to the 'post-war' peace in which problems emerge because the reality/normality changes. Aggression and anxiety, for example, which were experienced as 'normal' during the war, become 'intolerable', are experienced as extreme and appear out of proportion.

Dr Franciskovic presented a Pyramid of Intervention (Figure 16), illustrating how the needs of each individual change as the war is replaced by peace. At the outset of war, the most pressing form of aid is the provision of aid for basic needs for physical survival, such as food, blankets, plastic for windows, shelter and clothing. As the war continues, family groups, friends and communities, stretched beyond their limits are no longer able to provide adequate support, and external 'intervention' of emotional and psychological support can begin to play a part. It is during the 'post-war phase' that these 'psychological interventions', along with the economic input and the creation of new and re-establishment of old structures begin to be of greater importance in adapting to the new reality. In helping the community in this stage, Dr Franciskovic emphasised the need to take heed not to de-skill and disempower local professionals.

*Changes to the *identity of community*: due to refugees having a different influence in terms of street speech, type of music, smell of food, competition between refugees, displaced people and domicile for aid; changes to the *structure of communities*: due to demographic changes, domicile population feeling threatened, refugees seen as privileged, displaced people isolated, loss of solidarity; changes to *social institutions*: due to new rules and regulations, attempts to create new institutions, the process of privatisation, uneducated people taking up jobs.

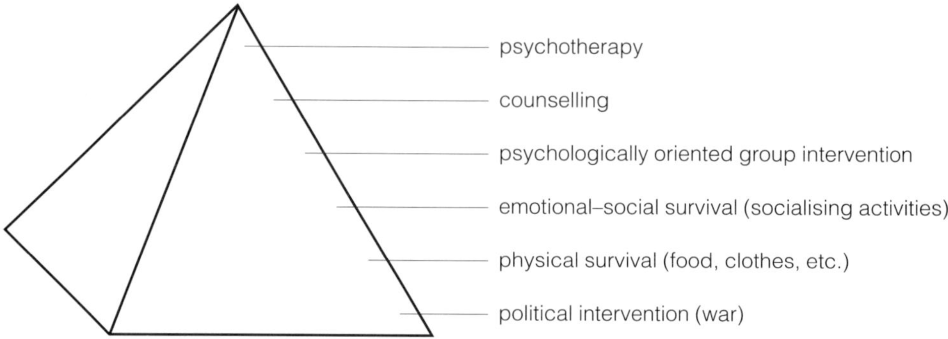

Figure 16. Pyramid of intervention (adaptation of pyramid used by Dr T Franciskovic in lecture)
By definition, the higher up the pyramid, the fewer people are reached

The art-making and art sessions offered in the pilot art therapy projects could be described in terms of Dr Franciskovic's pyramid as providing 'emotional–social and psychologically-oriented group intervention'. This was particularly useful in the context of refugee centres where individuals could find a 'socialising' structure in Dr Franciskovic's research ('socialising' was rated as the most useful intervention by refugees and displaced people). Group members can learn from their peers and support one another. Groups acted as little 'societies' in which the group could offer to individuals attention and inspiration. By being part of a group, individuals could be part of a process which involved movement and in which each person could watch others shift, change and transform their images – encouraging change in their own expression. In addition, the making of images in the presence of others could allow each person a voice through the image, which could be seen and heard.

From the above it is apparent that the art sessions offered different levels of intervention for different individuals; for most, providing an early sustaining and nourishing stage of the therapeutic process and for a few, the beginnings of insight-oriented therapy. As art therapists, the main objective was, and is, to be responsible as professionals to the individuals with whom we work. These responsibilities include acute awareness of the context, of the time-frame, of the level of vulnerability of the individuals, of the healthy elements, and an in-depth understanding and respect for the art process.

Implicit in a future art therapy service in a 'post-war phase' would be a 'psychologically-oriented intervention', where art therapy is a form of 'psychotherapy' in which the focus remains on the image and image-making in the presence of the art therapist. In addition, both professional and personal support to local carers and professionals would be fundamental in a future service, in the form of training, supervision, etc.

Pilot art therapy projects

Art therapy could be initiated in both Hrastnik and Prvic as a result of the stability that existed in Slovenia and Croatia respectively, despite the fact that the situation was, by definition, temporary.* Table 6 presents a bird's-eye view of both refugee centres during 1994 and responses to art sessions that took place.

*In contrast to this, in the context of Sarajevo and East Mostar individuals were daily exposed to danger and art therapy could not take place at that time.

	Hrastnik refugee centre	Prvic refugee centre
Aims	To observe informally the life and environment of the refugee centre, gradually to introduce art into the structures if appropriate and to assess the potential for art therapy	To increase ATI's understanding of art therapy work in the context of this war, to introduce art and to assess the potential for art therapy
Population	200: 107 children, 72 women, 21 men	24: 1 new-born, 9 children (aged 2–11), 11 adolescents, 3 women
Refugee average length of stay (at time of pilot project)	2 years	5 months
Existing support	No formal psychological support offered; permanent volunteers carrying out general support (practical and emotional)	1 psychologist and 1 teacher working as 'social worker', both part-time; centre officially overseen by Social Services, UNHCR, Split
Applicability of art sessions to culture	Art sessions congruous with the culture	Art sessions congruous with the culture
Time-frame of pilot projects	5 weeks: April–May 1994; 1 week: August 1994	17 days: October-November 1994
Overall response to art sessions	Immediacy of response: group art session environment enabled exploration of themes and concerns pertinent to each individual	Eager response to art sessions: group art session environment enabled exploration of themes and concerns pertinent to each individual
Space offered for art sessions	1st visit: art sessions took place in room also used as bedroom; 2nd visit: new hut offered appropriate space for art sessions; art sessions also took place outside	Art room offered at start of 3 weeks, 'removed' soon afterwards; all art sessions took place in dining room or outside thereafter
Interpreters	Volunteer provided interpreting where needed; otherwise interpreters not necessary at this stage	Most individuals spoke some English; interpreters not necessary at this stage
Art materials	International aid supplies ensured large quantities of basic art materials; in addition, ATI took specialist tools and materials unsure as to what was available	No art materials at the centre; all art materials and tools purchased by ATI locally

Table 6. **Summary of pilot art therapy projects at Hrastnik and Prvic refugee centres, 1994**

As summarised in the table above, it was possible for ATI to assess the practical considerations and obstacles relevant to planning and setting up a working model for an art therapy service in the context of the former Yugoslavia and, more generally, in situations of political conflict.

Setting up an art therapy service in the future:

In planning a working art therapy service (see p. 3, Model 1) a clear *structure* needs to be set up within which art therapy can take place. Through the two art therapy pilot projects and the interviews, it became apparent that it would be possible and appropriate to set up a structure for a functioning art therapy service in the former Yugoslavia.

1. In setting up an art therapy service, clarification from the outset of the parameters within which the work is to take place is essential.
Despite the fact that not all the (following) requirements were possible in the context of the refugee centres, a minimum 'requirement' was present – that of relative

stability – within the day-to-day lives of the refugees. Within this ATI could establish a reliable routine within the limitations of the time -frame and context, which were clarified at the outset.

2. The possibility of purchase of basic art materials locally would be important in the development of an art therapy service.
Basic art materials were available locally in Slovenia, Croatia and Bosnia and it was therefore possible to offer art sessions using local resources.

3. For an art therapy service to be implemented, a room/space would be necessary.
The physical space for offering art sessions in both refugee centres was limited. Adaptation to the restrictions presented by camp life and rules was necessary. It was as a result of art therapy training and consequent art therapy practice that the art-making could be contained, no matter where it took place: in the bedroom, in the dining room, on the hill, in the town dump.

4. Confidentiality: A space conducive to uninterrupted and confidential sessions would be necessary for the implementation of an art therapy service and for the art therapy work to be taken further.
Confidentiality could not be adhered to as most of the work took place in public spaces within the refugee centres.

5. For the implementation of an art therapy service it would be essential for art therapists to live separately from the centre in order to maintain therapeutic distance.
The fact that ATI members lived in the centres enabled useful and in-depth observation to be made which would have been difficult had ATI visited for the periods of the art sessions alone. However, this was not conducive to maintaining therapeutic distance.

6. In the implementation of an art therapy service the provision of interpreters would be necessary.
The use of interpreters was not necessary at this stage as many individuals spoke some English, or there was someone present within the group context able to translate where necessary, and the art images provided a central communication.

7. In the setting up of an art therapy service a referral system would need to be established.
In the context of the pilot art therapy projects, a referral system was not relevant.

8. In the implementation of an art therapy service the establishment of follow-up would be essential.
At Prvic refugee centre where local psychological support was already in place, there was a keen response to working alongside ATI, ensuring adequate follow-up and support for therapeutic work initiated, where necessary.

9. In implementing an art therapy service, collaboration with local psychological services would be essential and lead to the handing over of the service locally.
Working alongside local carers where possible was integral.

10. In setting up an art therapy service, support to local carers would be integral.
Offering professional and personal support to local carers was an identified need, in the pilot art therapy projects and the interviews.

11. Supervision for workers, and local carers (where appropriate), would be essential in setting up an art therapy service.
In both pilot projects, clinical supervision was not available.

12. Peer supervision and working in pairs would be essential tools in setting up an art therapy service.
Peer supervision was provided by ATI members working in pairs. This was both an effective means of support and a necessary tool in carrying out, monitoring and evaluating the therapeutic process.

13. In planning an art therapy service, consultation and follow-up supervision would be formalised and integral.
Consultation provided in London both before and after the three visits to the former Yugoslavia was essential.

Interviews

The interviews and meetings that took place in Croatia and Bosnia were extremely informative and crucial in establishing an adequate picture of existing therapeutic support, local needs and where and how to implement findings.

There are a number of reasons for the open-ended style of the interview and the consequent structure of the presentation of the information found: there was limited and inadequate written documentation on local services, statistics and other data. ATI met with as many organisations and individuals as was possible in the context of war and local circumstances. It was, however, usually impossible to arrange interviews beforehand due to the limited, or absence of, telephone/fax/postal facilities. In Bosnia, there did not appear to be much systematic planning and in many cases the style of aid inevitably evolved in response to the crisis. In East Mostar, for example, foreign aid and local services, where they existed, were disorganised. The Soros Foundation was in the early stages of gathering information, but at this stage it was still necessary to arrange on-the-spot meetings. In Croatia, reconstruction had started but insecurity continued to hamper progress. In addition to this, organisations were still in the process of establishing what was needed in the aftermath of the trauma of the war and with the crisis of displaced people and refugees.

It was not useful to pre-plan a set questionnaire in the UK when the situation in the former Yugoslavia was in flux. Despite this, a number of uniform questions remained a constant and were always asked:
- What psycho-social services do you offer?
- Do any psycho-social services you offer involve art, if so, in what context is art used?
- Do you know of any situations in which the arts are being used formally or informally?
- Do you know what art therapy is?
- In your experience, what is the response to and validity of therapy in general?
- Do you envisage art therapy as being relevant to the services provided by your organisation in this context?
- Could you detail the difficulties of setting up psycho-social support services?

The advantage of this interview process was that ATI was able to meet individuals and organisations face-to-face. It was the 'open-ended style' of the interview and attentive listening that yielded the most useful information. Responding to the needs of the context and not superimposing a pre-defined structure was one of ATI's main objectives.

ATI's findings are consistent with those of Dr Franciskovic as presented in 1996. In meetings in both Croatia and Bosnia, ATI found that economic resources and the local infrastructure were seriously depleted, the majority of professionals had left at the start of the war, the need for psychological support was growing daily and those local people taking up or thrown into the roles of caring were themselves 'burnt-out' and in urgent need of support and training. It was the international community that was looked to for provision of resources, professionals, psychological support and training. Along with this, emphasis was placed on the need for the international community to be sensitive to local needs and make provisions in direct response to these.*

In answer to the direct questions asked regarding art therapy and existing psycho-social questions, out of the 20 individuals and organisations interviewed the following are concluded:
- 17 thought that art therapy could provide a service that was not already offered
- 7 offered art projects (often informal); 2 offered 'art therapeutically'
- 13 saw a possibility of setting up an art therapy working structure within their existing service. (See Tables 1–4.)

No funding was available however and independent funding would have to be found.

Field-work

Field-work was an invaluable and integral aspect of ATI's work, as has been reiterated throughout this report. The method was merely to live in refugee centres, stay in Sarajevo and East Mostar, to try to live as the local people did, as far as possible, and through accumulating experience and often fortuitous moments of comprehension, in this way gain insight in to daily experiences and ways in which individuals were coping. Chance seemed to have played a large part in the circumstances which led to the results of this research and additional work.

A large and important part of ATI's role was ultimately to listen, night and day, to individual accounts of loss, pain, friendships, humour, love and humanity in people's day-to-day experience. ATI was witness to structures falling apart as well as to tremendous resilience.

---

*As an example: ATI was invited to attend a supervision session in Sarajevo by the International Rescue Committee (IRC). It was run for 15 counsellors working specifically with children. The request from these counsellors was for ATI as art therapists to accurately interpret children's drawings. There was a general misconception that one exact interpretation exists for a picture, and tremendous pressure was put on ATI to provide solutions, and make instant interpretations. The counsellors were working in the most difficult circumstances of ongoing war and appeared to be trying to grasp at something tangible, something 'factual', on which to hold. The images along with the 'specialists' from outside were expected to provide this.

In response to ATI's questions regarding art therapy, the following points emerged: art was already being used in the counselling work as a 'crude' diagnostic tool by untrained counsellors; educating the counsellors was of utmost importance as new traumas had been created in the clients attending counselling, resulting out of the lack of knowledge in the safe use of the art in the therapeutic process; art therapy would have a crucial role to play, both in direct work with children and in the training of counsellors.

A final word

ATI has attempted to describe fragments of art therapy at work and to assess what it could offer and why it took the form it did. ATI struggled with a desire to find solutions and solve problems while working in the context of war and so much suffering. Throughout the war in the former Yugoslavia, new non-government organisations were appearing, with experts, ideas and seminars, perhaps also attempting to find solutions. The majority offered vital support to the services set up by psychologists and teachers who stayed behind. Some of the enthusiasm has not developed further, and although local people reached out to organisations for training, manpower and resources, there was also a certain reserve and an expectation that what was being offered was simply rhetoric.

The research has been shaped, and is justified, by findings, detailed within 20 meetings, two pilot studies and field-work. The conclusions are clear: there is a place for both clinical art therapy input for children and adults and a pressing need for support and training of local carers and professionals.

PART III: PROJECT REPORT

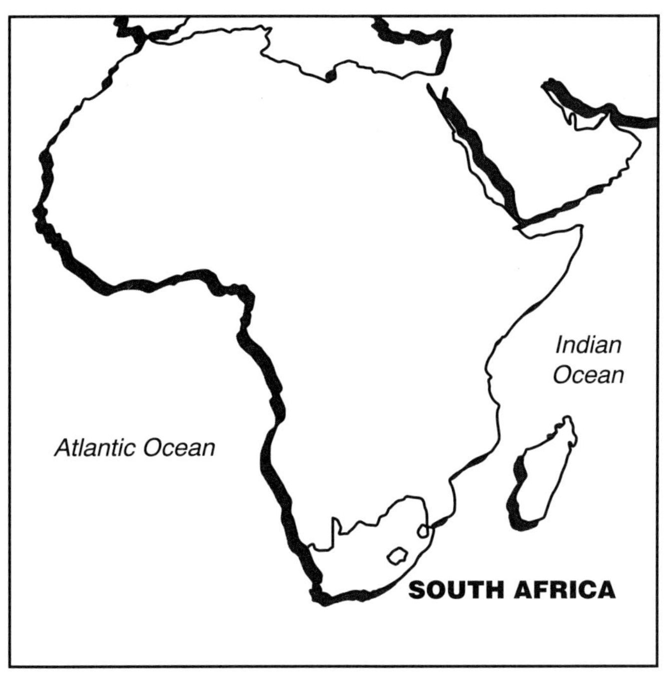

Art therapy workshops: KwaZulu–Natal, South Africa

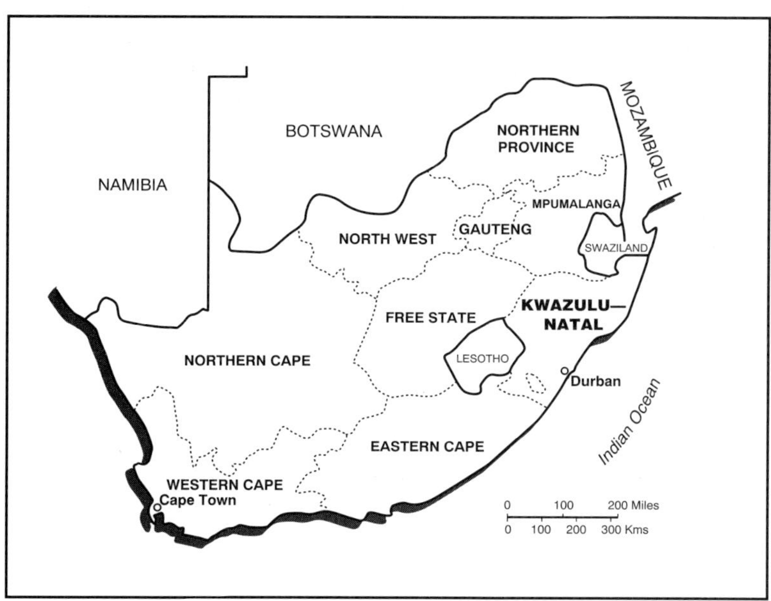

Figure 17. **Map of South Africa, 1996**

The Republic of South Africa 1996

Status	Republic
Area	1,220,845 sq km
	(471,369 sq miles)
Population	40,435,000
Capital	Pretoria (administrative)
	Cape Town (legislative)
Language	Afrikaans, English, various African languages
Religion	Christian majority, Hindu, Jewish and Muslim minorities
Currency	Rand (ZAR)
Organisations	Commonwealth, OAU, SADC, UN

Introduction

The following section is adapted from a report written for Dr N D Zuma, Minister of Health, South Africa, funders of the workshop and workshop participants. In contrast to Part II, this is not research but a report which documents and evaluates components that made up the workshop.

This report describes the 'Art Therapy Workshops', an intensive 4-week art therapy course for people working with children and adults who have directly experienced violence in KwaZulu–Natal. This idea was initiated in November 1994 by Liz Palmer of the Art Works Trust. The workshops took place in the Fine Art Department of the University of Durban–Westville (UDW), from 22 November to 16 December 1995 and were devised and run by two art therapists, Debra Kalmanowitz and Bobby Lloyd (ATI).

Initially, ATI were invited for one month to work directly with children in the townships of KwaZulu–Natal. However, they felt that in such a limited time-frame it would be of greater benefit to work with carers and professionals already working with children and adults in the community. This was due to time limits of the proposed work in relation to the specific situation in KwaZulu–Natal; the length of exposure to violence and the consequent level of 'trauma' experienced.

Also documented is the fact that care providers themselves are often burnt-out, overwhelmed and sorely lacking in training. ATI found that this was applicable to KwaZulu–Natal where it was evident that people were burdened and overwhelmed by huge workloads and a sense of the enormity of the problems. By offering carers some training they could acquire not only new skills but also take invaluable time in which to revitalise drained energies.

After a year of negotiations and local enquiry into this idea, the Fine Art Department of the University of Durban–Westville agreed to host the workshops. This corresponded with an initiative from Dr N D Zuma, Minister of Health, to the Committee of University Principals asking the committee to encourage universities to get involved in hospitals and health measures as part of a Community Outreach Programme. In addition, the Fine Art Department was already supporting a feasibility study for the proposed development of an art therapy course at UDW.

The workshop facilitators were accountable to the University of Durban–Westville and the Art Works Trust (both funding and organisational bodies).

KwaZulu–Natal

Natal has been and remains one of South Africa's most prosperous regions. The Zulu nation has survived as the largest and most nationalistic black group in South Africa. In the 1970s under apartheid large tracts of Zululand and Natal were designated part of the 'self-governing tribal homeland of KwaZulu' which has done much to promote Zulu nationalism. The Inkatha Freedom Party (IFP) won the provincial elections in 1994 and currently heads the provincial government. Violence still rages between supporters of the IFP and the African National Congress (ANC). At the regional level this violence is a result of many factors described below and at the national level the IFP and the ANC still have a fundamental disagreement over the level of independence of the provinces and the powers of the provincial government as enshrined in South Africa's new constitution.

'In much of KwaZulu–Natal there is an intermittent ongoing civil war. Part of the legacy of apartheid, its roots are in poverty, overcrowding, competition for limited jobs and resources, political rivalry. Crime and, increasingly, drug trafficking play a part. A generation has grown up accepting as the norm unacceptable levels of violence' (Art Works Trust, Appendix 5).

Durban, in the region of KwaZulu–Natal, is the third largest city, as well as the 'Asian capital' of South Africa. Despite being situated in KwaZulu the city has a predominantly white culture as well as mosques and bazaars taking up whole blocks of the city centre. The townships surrounding central Durban stretch for almost 20 miles and the main roads pass some of the worst poverty in southern Africa. Violent political events have not been a great feature in Durban life itself.

Despite the problems resulting from the abolition of apartheid and the accession of the ANC to government, the enormous goodwill of the South African people as a whole to make their new country work should not be underestimated.

The workshop

The workshop took place from Wednesday to Saturday over a four-week period. The participants were committed to attend each day for the full day from 8.30 am to 4.00 pm. On the Monday and Tuesday of each week, the facilitators visited areas in which participants worked in an attempt to gain greater understanding of the specifics of the situation in KwaZulu–Natal.

This four-week workshop was not a 'training' and therefore did not provide a qualification to practise as art therapists. However, it intended to provide participants with insights into the use of art in their work – drawing on each individual's intrinsic professional and academic knowledge and skills. The participants made a commitment to carry insights gained into their work as well as to pass these on to others working in the field.

The workshops were structured on an 'experiential' model (that is, learning by experiencing through doing) which is understood to be an effective way to teach about the process of art therapy.

Aims of the workshop

Three meetings were held at the Ecumenical Centre in Durban over the planning period, in the months prior to ATI's arrival. These were attended by fifteen to eighteen people representing different institutions and were called to discuss what individuals wanted from a course of this nature and what UDW could offer. A resulting list of expectations was used in formulating aims for the course. The aims were as follows:

1. To provide an intensive experience of art and art-making for participants as individuals and as part of a group which would hopefully lead to insights that would resonate in their work.

2. To provide a forum which would bring a wide concept of art and art therapy as a basis for continuing questioning with which participants can continue to work. These two aims were intended to contribute to:
- building confidence in using art materials and in the image-making process;
- a richer understanding of the potential of the different art media;
- a greater understanding of group-work and therapeutic group process;
- sensitivity to 'emotional indicators'; the use and limitations of interpretation of artwork;
- some understanding of principles, theory and application of art therapy.

3. To provide a forum in which the wealth of knowledge, skills and experience of participants could be shared.

4. To provide an opportunity for personal learning.

5. To define, with the participants, insights and skills learnt throughout the course. (These would be passed on to other workers and could be assimilated into their own work.)

The participants

There were nine participants. In planning the workshops there were two options concerning the choice of people to whom they should be offered:

The first option was to offer the workshops to people with some experience of working with mental health issues, but no formal training.

The second option was to offer them to people with some formal training in mental health issues and working in the field.

The second option was decided upon as it was felt that, for this training to have a longer on-going life, it would be beneficial for trained professionals to pass their insights on to workers in the field as well as use these insights in their work – given the time limits of the course.

The participants were a mixed ethnic group – five white and four black South Africans. For many of the participants, this was one of the first opportunities, post-apartheid, to come together for an extended workshop to work and think on an intense and personal level. The group consisted of two nurses, two counsellors, one educational psychologist, three clinical psychologists and one artist – ages ranging from 25–55. Except for one male nurse, all participants were female. This was a rich group with a wide range of experiences and skills whose sense of responsibility to pass on skills and insights added to their commitment, care, sensitivity, desire to learn, openness to personal risk-taking, honest communication, and willingness to form working relationships amongst themselves and to offer support.

All the participants were working with children and adults who have directly experienced violence in the region of KwaZulu–Natal in contexts such as schools and an orphanage in Durban, Imbali and Claremont townships and Kwa-Mashu squatter camp. The organisations with which they worked included the Medical Foundation for the Care of Victims, School Psychological Services, KwaZulu–Natal Survivors of Violence, Children and Violence in South Africa, Natal Society of Arts Outreach Programme and the University of Natal Department of Psychology. In general, all those who signed up were working at their fullest capacity, with few resources and looking to this training in the use of art as a means to enhance their work. Each participant already used art to a greater or lesser degree in their work and had observed its potential as a therapeutic tool. All were given time off from work to participate in this course (see Appendix 5).

In 1994, there were six trained art therapists in South Africa (there are presently more art therapists in training outside South Africa who intend to return with this training, but figures are unavailable). Even though art therapy is not currently recognised by the South African Medical and Dental Council, this is expected to change at some time in the future, especially now that ATASA (Art Therapy Association of South Africa) has been formally established (1996). Dr Zuma, the Minister for Health, has taken an interest in art therapy and therefore supported this project.

Workshop schedule

Times	Wednesday	Thursday	Friday	Saturday
8.30–9.30	Interactive art therapy group	Interactive art therapy group	Interactive art therapy group	Interactive art therapy group
9.30–10.00	Coffee	Coffee	Coffee	Coffee
10.00–12.00	Open studio	Materials workshop	Case conference	Open studio
12.00–1.30	Lunch	Lunch	Lunch	Lunch
1.30–3.30	Open studio	Articles discussion	Theme workshop	Seminar
3.30–4.00	Plenary	Plenary	Plenary	Plenary

Open art therapy studio
This studio space offered the opportunity for participants to work, in a group, at their own pace, on individual art-making (Fig. 18, Pl. 5).
Aim: To explore a wide range of art materials and enable immersion in the art-making process over an extended period of time. The 'art school art studio' atmosphere (contained by the therapeutic boundaries) aims to facilitate expression and foster creativity which encourages images to 'emerge'. It is with these images that the individual and the facilitator/therapist 'work'.

Interactive art therapy group
This group offered a 'non-directive' group art therapy experience.
Aim: To facilitate interpersonal learning – through the making of images – and to stimulate the creativity of the participants; to focus on group, rather than individual process. The model involves awareness of the group as a 'system' and willingness to use the social and cultural context of the group and its images as material for the group. Interaction between members and art materials is central.

Materials workshop
This workshop focused each week on a different material (clay, drawing, paint, scrap) (Fig. 19, Pl. 6).
Aim: To offer participants a chance to familiarise themselves with, and closely explore, the material in order to gain insight into its innate qualities and particular potential for emotional expression.

Theme workshop
This workshop focused each week on a different theme presented by the facilitators (Figs. 20 and 21, Pls. 7 and 8).
Aim: To offer participants a structured and focused art therapy experience in which a theme is provided and chosen in response to the themes and dynamic arising out of the group process.

Articles, seminars, case consultations
These different sessions were offered each week to provide an opportunity for
participants to bring their own case-work, as well as to discuss different topics,
articles given and questions arising.
Aim: To provide a forum for peer supervision (i.e. sharing professional knowledge
and insights gained in relation to particular cases presented); to relate theory to
participants' experience of the art; to provide a wider context for art and art therapy
in different settings and to open seminars to a wider interested audience.

Components of the workshop

Setting and space
The workshop was held in the first year Fine Art studio at UDW. The space provided
was most appropriate and excellent for the needs of the workshop – adequate light,
running water, storage space, wall space, tables, chairs, easels, toilet facilities. The fact
that it was an art studio enabled full use to be made of the art materials, e.g. washable
floors and walls.

In addition to the above, being on the university campus meant that there was the
luxury of access to a library, audio-visual equipment and administration office
(including photocopying machine and telephone).

The one disadvantage (which participants in this group were able to overcome
through their tenacity and commitment) was that the campus is physically set at a
distance from Durban, and difficult to reach – public transportation being infrequent.

Materials and equipment
The organisation, quantity , quality and variety of materials and equipment were
excellent, and greatly appreciated by both participants and facilitators. Some
materials were ordered from Johannesburg beforehand and were available at the
start of the workshop. Scrap materials were collected by participants and were
integral.

General administration
Most of the administration was organised prior to the facilitators' arrival by the
first-year Fine Art Lecturer. This solid groundwork facilitated smooth running of the
course. On leave of absence in the UK, she set up an administrative support system
for the workshop which included the Fine Art department secretary for general
administration; a Fine Arts student as an assistant with photocopying and general
duties; and the Fine Art department technician for provision and maintenance of
materials and equipment.

Day-to-day administration
There was no centralised responsibility on site which resulted in the burden of work
falling upon the assistant. Although the student/assistant worked over and above
her brief she did not have the authority or knowledge to liaise with management etc.
This could be avoided in the future by the allocation of clear responsibility with
identified channels of communication.

Funding
This was the responsibility of two bodies and adequately covered all needs:

1. The Art Works Trust provided salaries (including research and preparation) in the UK.
2. UDW covered personal expenses including accommodation; car rental and petrol allowance; consultancy fees and all workshop costs including materials, administration, photographic documentation.

Visits
Part of the facilitators' role was to visit participants' places of work. Although it was not possible to visit all work settings, the visits were fundamental to the facilitators' understanding of context; also to later discussions in the workshops of ways in which art therapy insights could fit into the individual work settings.

Summary

The course structure succeeded in enabling participants to grasp basic principles in the use of art in a healing capacity. This was apparent throughout the course and in the comments made in the evaluation. Based on their experience of the different structures of the experiential workshops the participants appeared to grasp the principles of art therapy: they began to question and assess the different applications of art therapy in their various settings and the possibility of adapting the insights to different needs and situations. For example : applying art-making (not art therapy per se) in community settings and the value this would serve.

Integral to the learning was the acknowledgement of the brevity of the course and its limits. The focus in discussing the application of art therapy (towards the end of the four weeks) was on what the participants had learned and could implement rather than what they could not learn in such a short period. The focus was also on ways in which individuals could work at their own level – integrating new insights into their previous knowledge and skills.

At the start of the course there was an expression of the unfamiliarity with a 'non-directive experiential' method of teaching. There was an expectation that the teaching would take the form of lectures by the facilitators. A non-directive method of teaching is in contrast to the more directive approach which dominates the South African education system. There was also a curious interest in the idea of 'arts therapy', but a general difficulty in conceiving how it could work.

Gradually, through their participation in the course, these expectations were replaced by involvement in both the group and the art-making process. Daily, the workshop was filled with a rich and complex expression of each individual's personal experience and the conflict and frustrations of living and working in South Africa at this time. The willingness to face each other with an openness and to bring, listen and work with their past and present as white and black South Africans contributed to an intense and moving workshop.

Certain themes and issues were particularly central and are included here as an indication of the spirit of the workshop. There was continuing discussion concerning the contrast between traditional forms of healing and western forms of counselling and how each individual negotiated a balance.

At different times most participants expressed their sense of homelessness and at the same time their strong sense of belonging. Both black and white participants appeared to be in the process of negotiating for themselves a place in the new reality.

The art-work and the group process often appeared to reflect a microcosm of South Africa as it appears at this time, where the general climate in South Africa is one of acceptance and reconciliation. As individuals, working independently on their own art process, there was an openness to share personal stories that concerned both the past and the present. As a group however, art-work clearly reflected a denial of difference and a desire to create a sense of harmony.

All the participants felt overwhelmed by the lack of facilities, the extent of the problem and their personal workloads. There was a tremendous sense of guilt amongst the participants that this workshop was proving useful on a personal level and that they were taking time away from work to gain new skills.

Throughout the course, a strong group dynamic evolved. From a group of professionals who had come from different backgrounds and experiences, with each individual containing his/her own diverse expectations and mixed emotions, developed a learning group with growing motivation to absorb as much as possible for application back into their work/lives. In addition, they gradually became a more cohesive unit with much potential for mutual support and encouragement – able to acknowledge differences and work with that which they could share.

The following are comments made in the final case conference/supervision session, demonstrating immediate responses and individual's understanding of their experience of the workshops:

'When I was doing art I was not talking but in that silence my capacity to listen was greatly improved.'

'It evoked feelings in me. As I put it down I came up with very strong feelings I was unaware of . . . I thought I would be directed and judged. I put the pain down on the paper. I deal with my anger differently.'

'It relaxes me so much. In the relaxing things emerge.'

'I have learned about holding on, letting things happen, rather than jumping in, about letting the struggle go on, about trusting and restraint.'

'I will take away two goals: I learned the importance of respecting the art-work. I would like to awaken people to the power and creativity that is already there; to give people the experience to talk about inner things in a safe environment and finding a source of inner strength. There is light and colour and not just darkness – potential of the inner world.'

'I am aware I can be my own healer. I can integrate the elements, lose them and get there again.'

'It gives people a place in which to talk about feelings. It is a safe place, made possible by the group.'

'The idea of "witness" interests me – the quiet unconditional witnessing of someone else's story and the power this can hold. This can be applied to our work.'

'It works on different levels. If all we do is provide a safe place for people to come, at least they can know that somebody will be there for them.'

By the end of the workshops, it was apparent that individuals were beginning to assimilate the basic principles of art in therapy and had begun to develop ideas of how to include art in their work. As a group they formalised a first date to meet and make plans for implementing their insights.

Monitoring methods for evaluation

Documentation
All art-work was documented through slides and/or photographic film.

Process notes
All workshops and groups were recorded by the facilitators through process notes.

Questionnaires
These were confidential questionnaires handed out and filled in on the first day of the course (see Appendix 7).

Evaluations
These were also confidential, handed out and filled in on the last day of the course (see Appendices 8 and 9).

Long-term evaluations
These were required from participants by UDW one year after the workshops took place.

Supervision
This took two forms:
– London-based, for a three-month period before the workshops with a senior art therapist; used by the facilitators in devising and structuring the course, and on their return in evaluating it.
– Throughout the course, in the form of peer supervision between the facilitators, to monitor the progress of the workshops, and offer support and guidance.

Evaluation

On the final day of the course, the participants were asked to fill out an evaluation form and they were invited to carefully examine and candidly assess the course. For each component and for the course overall they were asked to appraise the effectiveness and relevance to their learning; evaluated on a 5-point scale with 5 as a very high appraisal and 1 as very low. The overall evaluation for the course was 4.9, with the experiential workshops achieving 4.3 and the discussion groups achieving 3.9 (see Appendix 9).

Based on this point method and on questions answered, overall it would seem the workshops and discussion groups were effective and relevant to each individual's needs both professionally and personally. The experiential groups were found to be the most useful despite unfamiliarity with the method of teaching. The discussion groups and seminars brought a range of reactions. Generally there was a desire for the facilitators to provide 'facts and figures'. The facilitators understood this request, but felt it was essential to balance this with the wider principle from which they could later draw as opposed to providing a solution to a particular problem. They also felt that their role as both facilitators and seminar group leaders was vast and the workshop could therefore benefit from different professional input. In the light of this, it would be effective to include guest lecturers in the seminar slot.

Written material and handouts were thought to be comprehensive and informative. It could be seen that art therapy can be applied and used responsibly in the different settings according to each individual's personal knowledge and level at which he or she works.

Proposals for the future

- Participants to divide into pairs and to work together to introduce art into their different work situations. The pair-work was suggested for support, sharing of knowledge and peer supervision.
- Regular group meetings – beginning February 1996. These were suggested to offer support and to carry on the momentum.
- Collaboration with local artists in order to implement insights/skills: the artists and group members working together to offer art therapeutically.

'Expanding Circles'

These could be based on a scheme successfully utilised in follow-up to a training seminar in Israel offered to stress-workers from the former Yugoslavia. The 'Expanding Circles' would involve subsequent follow-up in-country training workshops instructed by the participants, *and closely supervised by the facilitators (or prepared with their help)*. The workshops would take the form of small seminars in which the material learned would be shared with a broader circle of local workers (Dr Reuven Gal (1995) in *Helping the Helpers*).

Conclusion

The project described here is by no means a revolutionary idea. The concept is based on well-known principles of training as used in a variety of different settings by art therapists as well as other health practitioners. Seminars such as the Helping the Helpers project referred to in this report offered an invaluable example and gave courage in the planning stages. What was unique was that this was the first intensive art therapy workshop in KwaZulu–Natal: offering workshops in the use of art which intended not only to lead to insights which could be assimilated into participants' work and passed on to others, but also to replenish depleted energy.

In offering experiential workshops as a learning model the demystifying of a process was possible and this made for a very real and human exchange. It is hoped that through this course the participants will have been able to strengthen and deepen not only their knowledge, insights and skills, but also their motivation to persist – in the face of the continuing burden of their work with those who have experienced violence in KwaZulu–Natal.

Update 1996

The following update was received on 7 March 1996 from the participants of the workshop who have formed a group with the working title, the Art Therapy Group.*

This group of people has decided to meet regularly to help in using the skills gained at the workshop. Regular meetings help in supporting each other in getting this kind of work more known. In addition to this they are working together on several pilot projects in which making art is used as the primary therapy. These pilot projects include: 'art therapy' training for the educare workers active in the area of Shobashobane where the Christmas Day killings took place, including both Inkatha Freedom Party and African National Congress areas; therapy groups with flood survivors in Pietermaritzburg, through Midlands Hospital; art therapy work with young groups in Inanda; and work with youth leaders in Clermont.

*The ATG do not practise art therapy but use art in a therapeutic capacity within their work.

Glossary

The following definitions relate specifically to terms used in the text of this document. As such, they are defined by ATI in this context.

ANC African National Congress

Apartheid Afrikaans word for apartness or separation. The word is Afrikaans (the South African language derived from Dutch) for apartness or separation, officially used in South Africa from 1948 and enforced by law, applying segregation between black and white South Africans.

ARC American Refugee Committee

Art sessions In an art session the art-making is perceived as therapeutic but does not imply the discipline of clinical art therapy practice. The art-making is allied to artistic expression and therefore although therapeutic implies different parameters. Art sessions do not rely on previous art skills.

Art therapy Art therapy is a form of psychotherapy. In an art therapy session the individual is invited to draw, paint, sculpt. The focus in art therapy is on the image and the image-making in the presence of the therapist. At its centre is the understanding that this process can lead to change. Art therapy does not rely on previous art skills.

Art therapist The art therapist is a trained professional, with a minimum of a postgraduate training or master's degree in art therapy and an initial degree in art or another relevant degree such as psychology. Individuals must have obtained relevant work experience in the caring field before entry into an art therapy training and must show a continuing commitment to personal art processes.

ATASA Art Therapy Association of South Africa

ATI Art Therapy Initiative

BAAT British Association of Art Therapists

Catharsis The discharge or purging of emotion enabled by expression, for example, or by abreaction (the free expression and release of a previously repressed emotion).

Closed art therapy group A closed group is run at the same time on a regular basis for individuals who are referred. The group is closed to others and therefore the membership remains constant. In this group a 'group culture' can develop and trust can be established. The individual can therefore gain from both the art process and the group process and the therapeutic work has potential to be developed in greater depth.

Conscious In psychoanalytic theory mental activity can take place in two modes, one conscious, the other unconscious. Conscious mental activity is what one is immediately aware of, knows and works through thought processes.

Consultation The act of consulting to seek specialist opinion, advice, information.

Consultant Specialist who offers professional opinion/advice on his/her area of expertise.

Containing Holding of another person's difficult feelings which are otherwise uncontained. A type of holding – such as a mother may give to her distressed child. In psychoanalytic theory this term is used to describe the way in which one person can contain/hold and understand another's experience.

Creativity The ability to bring something new into existence. The capacity to arrive at novel but valid solutions to problems. The capacity to create imaginative products which are compelling.

Feedback Feedback is the process through which the individual can discover how well his/her behaviour, as perceived by others, corresponds to his/her intentions. This takes the form of direct mutual communication. This is essential for effective training and helping.

IFP Inkatha Freedom Party

Image The images or pictures made in an art therapy session are seen as forms of, for example, imaginations, dreams, cognitions, thoughts, beliefs, memories and feelings. The images hold many meanings and generate multiple interpretations. These can be reflected upon in depth and emphasis is placed on the meaning the individual gives to his/her image. The image is not judged for technical or aesthetic competence.

Interpretation Expounding the meaning of (dreams, images, pictures, words), explaining, understanding the meaning of in a specified manner, making out or bringing out the meaning of.

IRC International Rescue Committee

Open art therapy group The open group is run regularly at the same time for any individual who chooses to join or is referred. In this group the membership is constantly changing and the therapeutic benefits of the group such as sharing and trust are sometimes not possible.

PAC Pan African Congress

Post traumatic stress disorder (PTSD) The essential feature of this disorder is the development of the characteristic symptoms following a psychologically distressing event that is outside the range of usual human experience (i.e. outside the range of such common experiences as simple bereavement, chronic illness, business losses, and marital conflict). The stressor producing this syndrome would be markedly distressing to almost anyone, and is usually experienced with intense fear, terror, and helplessness. The characteristic symptoms involve re-experiencing the traumatic event, avoidance of stimuli associated with the event or numbing of general responsiveness, and increased arousal. The diagnosis is not made if the disturbance lasts less than one month.

The most common traumata involve either a serious threat to one's life or physical integrity; a serious threat or harm to one's children, spouse, or other close relatives or friends; sudden destruction of one's home or community; or seeing another person who has recently been, or is being, seriously injured or killed as a result of an accident or physical violence. In some cases the trauma may be learning about a serious threat or harm to a close friend or relative, e.g. that one's child has been kidnapped, tortured or killed. (*Diagnostic and statistical manual of mental disorders* 3rd ed.)

Psychology The science of the mind, but also the science of behaviour. Specialists may be qualified in one branch of the subject, e.g. child, clinical, abnormal, educational; or in a particular system of thought, e.g. Gestalt, Jungian, Freudian.

Psychologist A person trained in any form of psychology.

Psychotherapy The clinical practice of healing the mind. Psychotherapy may be either individual or group, superficial or deep. It can have different intentions, being either interpretative, supportive or suggestive, and can be based in a particular system of thought, e.g. Jungian, Freudian. It examines past and present concerns and encourages the person to understand themselves better.

Psychotherapist A person who practises psychotherapy, of any school, who could have a medical or lay background and who has received a training from a recognised institution.

Referral procedure The system by which an individual is forwarded for therapeutic support. This can be from any individual or department, for example teacher, social worker, psychologist, nursing staff, family or self-referral.

Repression The process by which an unacceptable idea or impulse to action is made unconscious.

SACP South African Communist Party

Supervision Supervision is a working alliance between a supervisor and a worker or workers in which the worker can reflect on him/herself in his/her working situation. This is achieved by giving an account of his/her work and receiving feedback and where appropriate, guidance and appraisal. The object of this alliance is to maximise the competence of the worker in providing a helping service.

Therapy The process of treating or healing or curing.

Therapeutic boundaries This refers to the contract between the therapist and the individual and concerns the limits and boundaries of the session and the therapy. This includes the space, length of session, the time of the session each week, the time span of the therapy, confidentiality, safe-keeping of images, consistency and reliability of the therapist, the relationship and the session. These therapeutic boundaries enable safety and trust to be developed.

Trauma This refers to a completely unexpected experience which the individual is unable to assimilate. When it happens, the immediate response to psychological trauma is shock. The individual might either recover spontaneously or develop a neurosis because defences come into play and try to repress the experience.

Unconscious In psychoanalytic theory mental activity can take place in two modes, one conscious, the other unconscious. Unconscious mental activity refers to processes of which one is not aware but can affect behaviour. Some unconscious processes can become conscious easily but some are subject to repression.

UNHCR United Nations High Commission for Refugees

UNICEF United Nations Children's Fund

Bibliography

Art therapy

Allan, John (1988) *Inscapes of the Child's World: Jungian Counselling in Schools and Clinics*. Dallas, Texas: Spring Publications, Inc.

Dalley, T. and Case, C. (1994) *The Handbook of Art Therapy*. London: Routledge .

Dileo, J. (1983) *Interpreting Children's Drawings*. New York: Brunner/Mazel.

Furth, G. M. (1988) *The Secret World of Drawings: Healing through Art*. Boston: Sigo Press.

Kramer, E. (1993) *Art as Therapy with Children*. Rev. ed. Chicago: Magnolia.

Kwiatowska, H. (1978) *Family Therapy and Evaluation Through Art*. Springfield: Charles. C. Thomas.

Levine, E. (1995) *Tending the Fire: Studies in Art, Therapy and Creativity*. Toronto: Palmerston Press.

Liebmann M. (ed.) (1994) *Art Therapy with Offenders*. London and Bristol, Pennsylvania: Jessica Kingsley Publishers.

McNiff, Shaun (1992) *Art as Medicine: Creating a Therapy of the Imagination*. Boston: Shambala.

McNiff, Shaun (1981) *The Arts and Psychotherapy*. Springfield, Illinois: Charles C. Thomas, Publishers.

Moon, Bruce (1987) *Existential Art Therapy*. Springfield, Illinois: Charles C. Thomas, Publishers.

Naumberg, M. (1995) *Dynamically Oriented Art Therapy*. Chicago: Magnolia.

Rhyne, J. (1984) *The Gestalt Art Experience*. Chicago, Illinois: Magnolia Street Publishers.

Robbins, A. (1984) *The Artist as Therapist*. New York: Human Sciences Press Inc.

Rubin, J.A. (ed.) (1987) *Approaches to Art Therapy: Theory and Technique*. New York: Brunner/Mazel.

Schaverien, Joy (1992) *The Revealing Image: Analytical Art Psychotherapy in Theory and Practice*. London, New York: Routledge.

Waller, D. (1993) *Group Interactive Art Therapy: its use in Training and Treatment*. London: Routledge.

Art and creativity

Eliade, M. (1992) *Symbolism, the Sacred, and the Arts*. New York: Continuum.

Fuller, P. (1980) *Art and Psychoanalysis*. London: Writers and Readers Press.

Fuller, P. (1983) *The Naked Artist: Art and Biology*. London: Writers and Readers Press.

Kellogg, R. (1970) *Analysing Children's Art*. Mountain View, Ca: Mayfield Publishing Company.

Lewis, P. (1993) *Creative Transformation: The Healing Power of the Art*. Wilmette, Illinois: Chiron Publications.

Lowenfeld, V. (1970) *Creative and Mental Growth*. 5th edn. New York: Macmillan.

Milner, M. (1981) *On Not Being Able to Paint*. 5th edn. London: Heinemann Educational (first published 1950).

Storr, A. (1975) *The Dynamics of Creation*. London: Penguin.

Expressive arts therapies

Jennings, S. and Minde, A. (1990) *Art Therapy and Drama Therapy: Their Relation and Practice*. London: Jessica Kingsley Publishers.

Knill, Paolo J., Nienhaus Barba, H. and Fuchs, M. (1995) *Minstrels of Soul: Intermodal Expressive Therapy*. Toronto: Palmerston Press.

Lewis, P. (1984) *Theoretical Approaches in Dance Movement Therapy*. Vols I and II. Dubuque, Iowa: Kendal-Hunt.

Priestley, M. (1975 and 1984) *Music Therapy in Action*. London: Constable.

Further reading

Casement, P. (1985) *On Learning From the Patient*. London: Routledge.

Cooper, J.C. (1978) *An Illustrated Encyclopaedia of Traditional Symbols*. London: Thames and Hudson Ltd.

Frankl, Victor E. (1984) *Man's Search for Meaning*. London, New York: Washington Square Press.

Hillman, J. (1978) *The Myth of Analysis*. New York: Harper and Row.

Hillman, J. (1977) *Re-Visioning Psychology*. New York: Perennial Library.

Levine, S.K. (1992) *Poiesis: The Language of Psychology and the Speech of the Soul*. Toronto: Palmerston Press.

Lomas, P. (1992) *The Limits of Interpretation: What's wrong with Psychoanalysis?* London: Penguin.

Moore, T. (1989) *Blue Fire: Selected Writings by James Hillman*. New York: Harper and Row.

Rank, Otto (1968) *Art and Artist; Creative Urge and Personality Development*. New York: Agathon Press.

Watkins, M. (1990) *The Development of Imaginal Dialogues: Invisible Guests*. Boston, Massachusetts: Sigo Press.

Yalom, I. D. (1985) *The Theory and Practic of Group Psychotherapy*. (3rd edn.) New York: Basic Books Inc.

Other classics include: Freud, Jung, Klein, Rogers, Moustakas, Axline, Winnicott.

Journals

Inscape, the Journal of the British Association of Art Therapists, obtainable from BAAT, 11a Richmond Road, Brighton, BN2 3RL.

The American Journal of Art Therapy, (published in association with the American Art Therapy Association), obtainable from Vermont College of Norwich University, Montpelier, Vermont 05602, USA.

The Arts in Psychotherapy, an International Journal, obtainable from Elsevier Science, Boulevard, Langford Lane, Kidlington, Oxford OX5 1GB.

Related reading: Former Yugoslavia and South Africa

Aga Khan, Sadruddin; Bib Talal, Hassan (1986) *The Dynamics of Displacement: a Report for the Independent Commission on International Humanitarian Issues.* Zed Books.

Ayalon, Ofra (1992) *Rescue: Community Oriented Preventive Education for Coping with Stress.* Haifa, Israel: Chevron Publishing, Word Publications.

Bunjevac, Tomislav and Kuterovac, Gordana (June 1994) *Report on the Results from a Psychological Screening of School Age Children in Herzegovina.* Zagreb, Croatia: Department of Psychology, Faculty of Philosophy, University of Zagreb.

Chichester, David (1992) *Shots in the Street: Violence and Religion in South Africa.* Cape Town: Oxford University Press.

Fraser, M. (1974) *Children in Conflict.* London: Penguin.

Garcia Del Soto, A. G. (September 1994) *Zbirni Center Hrastnick: A Pyychological Description of a Refugee Centre in Slovenia.* Unpublished.

Glenny, Misha (1993) *The Fall of Yugoslavia: The Third Balkan War.* London: Penguin Books.

Hunter, Brian (ed.) (1996) *The Statesman's Year-Book: a Statistical, Political and Economic Account of the States of the World for the Year 1996–1997.* London and Basingstoke: Macmillan Press.

Isaacson, Rupert (1995) *South Africa, Swaziland and Lesotho.* London: Cadogan Books.

Lapping, Brian (1986) *Apartheid: a History.* London: Grafton Books.

Malcolm, Noel (1994) *Bosnia – A short History.* London: Macmillan Papermac.

Mandela, Nelson (1994) *Long Walk to Freedom: the Autobiography of Nelson Mandela.* New York and London: Little, Brown.

Medact Group Action Report (1994) Traumatised Children in former Yugoslavia. *Medact Global Security Magazine* (Summer), p. 12.

Mooli, L. and Cohen, A. (eds) (1993) *Community Stress Prevention.* Volume 2. Israel: The Community Stress Prevention Centre.

Omladinski Pamphlet (1994) Mostar. Unpublished.

Sogoric, Selma (1992) War in Croatia. *Medact Global Security Magazine* (Spring), pp. 4–5.

Straker, Gill (1992) *Faces in the Revolution: The Psychological Effects of Violence on Township Youth in South Africa.* Capetown: David Philip.

UNHCR (1993) *The State of the World's Refugees 1993: The Challenge of Protection.* London: Penguin Books.

UNICEF (1994a) *Report on War Trauma Among Children in Sarajevo – February 1994.* Unicef: Emergency Operations in former Yugoslavia: Reports 1994. New International Publications.

UNICEF (1994b) *Library Project Report – Croatia – Presentation to Art Therapy Conference.* Ferrara, Italy – September, 1994. Unpublished.

UNICEF (1996) *The State of the World's Children 1996.* Oxford: Oxford University Press.

Van Rusburg, H. J. (ed.) (1995) *South African Year Book 1995.* South Africa: South Africa Communication Service.

Van der Veer, Guus (1992) *Counselling and Therapy with Refugees: Psychological Problems of Victims of War, Torture and Repression.* New York: John Wiley.

Vulliamy, Ed (1994) *Seasons in Hell: Understanding Bosnia's War*. London and New York: Simon and Schuster.

Winn, Linda (1994) *Post Traumatic Stress Disorder and Dramatherapy: Treatment and Risk Reduction*. London: Jessica Kingsley Publishers.

Related articles

Callaghan, K. (1993) Movement Psychotherapy with Adult Survivors of Political Torture and Organised Violence. *The Arts in Psychotherapy* **20**:411–21.

Dermen, Sira (1990) *A Psychotherapist in Armenia,* paper given to the Applied Section of the British Psycho-analytical Society, September 26th, 1990.

Gal, Dr Reuven (May 1995) 'Helping the Helpers': Training Seminars in Israel to stress-relief workers from the former Yugoslavia, Israel. Unpublished.

Gersie, A. (1995) Arts Therapies Practice in Inner City Slums: Beyond the Installation of Hope. *The Arts in Psychotherapy* **22**:207–15.

Gibson, K. (1989) Children in Political Violence. *Society, Science, Medicine* **28**(7):659–67.

Golub D. (1984) Symbolic Expression in Post-Traumatic Stress Disorder: Vietnam Combat Veterans in Art Therapy. *The Arts in Psychotherapy* **12**:285–96.

Gregorian, V., Azarian, A., De Maria, M. and McDonald, L. (1996) Colours of Disaster: The Psychology of the 'Black Sun'. *The Arts in Psychotherapy* **23**(1).

Hanes, Michael J. (1995) Utilizing Road Drawings as a Therapeutic Metaphor in Art Therapy. *American Journal of Art Therapy* **34** (August).

Horowitz, M.J. Comprehensive Analysis of Change after Brief Dynamic Psychotherapy. *American Journal of Psychiatry* **143**:5.

Howard, R. (1990) Art Therapy as an Isomorphic Intervention in the Treatment of a Client with post-traumatic Stress Disorder. *The American Journal of Art Therapy* **28**:79–86.

Johnson, D.R. (1987) The Role of the Creative Arts Therapies in the Diagnosis and Treatment of Psychological Trauma, *The Arts in Psychotherapy* **14**:7–13.

Kalmanowitz, D. and Lloyd, B. (1997) Fragments of Art at Work: Art Therapy in the former Yugoslavia. Unpublished article.

Klingman A., Koenigsfeld E. and Markman D. (1987) Art Activity with Children Following Disaster: a Preventive-oriented Crisis Intervention Modality. *The Arts in Psychotherapy* **14**:153–66.

Learmonth, M. (1994) Witness and Witnessing in Art Therapy. *Inscape* **1**:19–22.

Lifton, R.J. and Olson, Eric (76) The Human Meaning of Total Disaster: The Buffalo Creek Experience. *Psychiatry* **39** (February).

Melzak, S. (1992) Secrecy, Privacy, Survival, Repressive Regimes, and Growing Up. *Bulletin of the Anna Freud Centre* **15**:205–24.

Melzak, S. and Woodcock, Jeremy (1991) Child Refugees Who are Survivors of Repression and its Concomitants, Including Torture. *Association for Child Psychology and Psychiatry*, London, Occasional Paper, No. 6.

Tony Smythe and Nick Lewer (1992) Yugoslavia, (Page 3); Selma Sogoric: War in Croatia, (Pages 4–5): *Medact Global Security Magazine* (Spring).

Modric, Zlatan (1994) Trauma and Reality. Video-Film Serial Document, Croatia. Unpublished.

Ochberg, F.M. and Fojtik, K.M. (1984) A Comprehensive Mental Health Clinical Service Program for Victims: Clinical issues and therapeutic strategies. *American Journal of Social Psychiatry* **4**(3):12–19.

Sanderson M. (1995) Art Therapy with Victims of Torture: A New Frontier. *Canadian Art Therapy Journal* **9**:1.

Seligman Z. (1991) Trauma and Drama: A Lesson from the Concentration Camps. *The Arts in Psychotherapy* **22**(2):119–32.

Smythe, Tony and Lewer, Nick (1992) Yugoslavia. *Medact Global Security Magazine* (Spring), p. 3.

Stronach-Buschel, B. (1990) Trauma, Children, and Art. *Amerian Journal of Art Therapy* **29**:48–52.

Swartz, Leslie and Levett, Ann (1989) Political Repression and Children in South Africa: The Social Construction of Damaging Effects. *Society, Science, Medicine* **28**:741–50.

Terr, Lenore C. (1980) Forbidden Games: Post-Traumatic Child's Play. *Journal of the American Academy of Child Psychiatry* **20**:741–60.

Appendices

Appendix 1: UNICEF Mostar psycho-social survey of children

Results of war trauma screening
- 85 per cent of children have been forced to leave their town or village during war.
- 57 per cent of children reported that one or both of their parents were wounded.
- 19 per cent have been injured.
- 19 per cent have siblings that have been injured.
- 62 per cent have seen dead bodies.
- 90 per cent have seen someone who was injured in the war.
- 95 per cent have been in a situation during the war in which they thought they would be killed.
- 100 per cent of children have experienced shelling very nearby.
- 75 per cent have had their homes attacked or shelled.
- 67 per cent had been shot at by snipers.
- 43 per cent have experienced serious food and water shortage.
- 24 per cent reported they thought they would die from the cold.

Trauma reactions
Results show that frequently:
- 53 per cent of children think life is not worth living.
- 71 per cent have terrifying dreams.
- 77 per cent have experienced stomach aches; this may be evidence of extreme hunger, or may be psycho-somatically conditioned.

Note: data were collected from a random sample of 21 children (9 boys and 12 girls, from 12 to 17 years old) living in East Mostar in January 1994. The sample was relatively small due to extreme security conditions.

Appendix 2: UNICEF Step-by-Step to Recovery programme

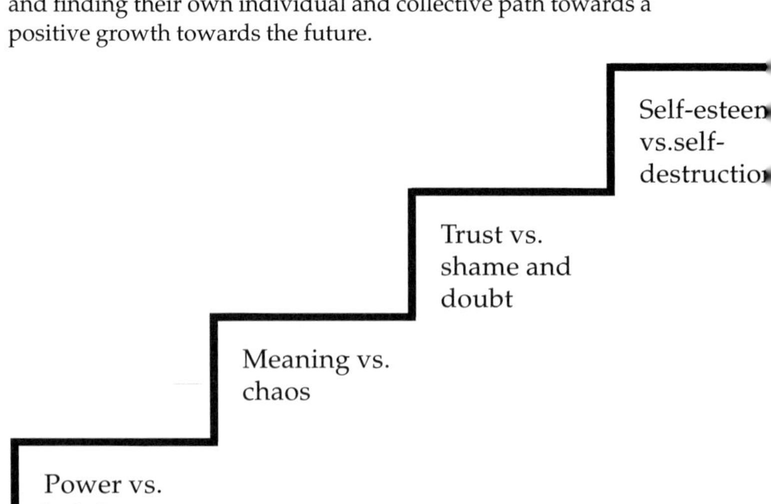

With 1995 drawing to a close, the UNICEF funded multi-media psycho-social programme 'Step-by-Step to Recovery', held during the course of the year, in libraries Croatia wide, has become a focal point for children traumatised by war. It has become their voice; a collection of stories, poems and drawings in which children have expressed their greatest joys, their deepest fears and a vision of how they see their future.

The project which began in 1993, was initiated by well-known art therapist and psychologist Dr Arpad Barath, a member of the Institute of Psychology, at Zagreb's Medical University. The concept involves using the library environment as the most conducive setting for art therapy work with children. The project incorporates the use of psychological discussions and games, drama and puppet therapy, computer games, art and writing therapy.

This year, the project involved 22 libraries, in 14 cities throughout Croatia, with some 2732 children participating. Librarians, pedagogues, teachers and psychologists worked with children, most refugee and displaced, helping them express their post-traumatic stress and negative emotions and transform them into creative works. The results achieved were inspiring.

Children delighted in the opportunity to have a voice, a medium to express themselves, even the most withdrawn. Many of them introverted, anxious, suffering from shock and anti-social behaviour at the beginning of the programme, truly found peace and expression by the end of the therapy. The creative process (picture below), facilitated by a series of 12-step psychological and creative techniques, led the children to problem-solving, recognising and developing their goals and finding their own individual and collective path towards a positive growth towards the future.

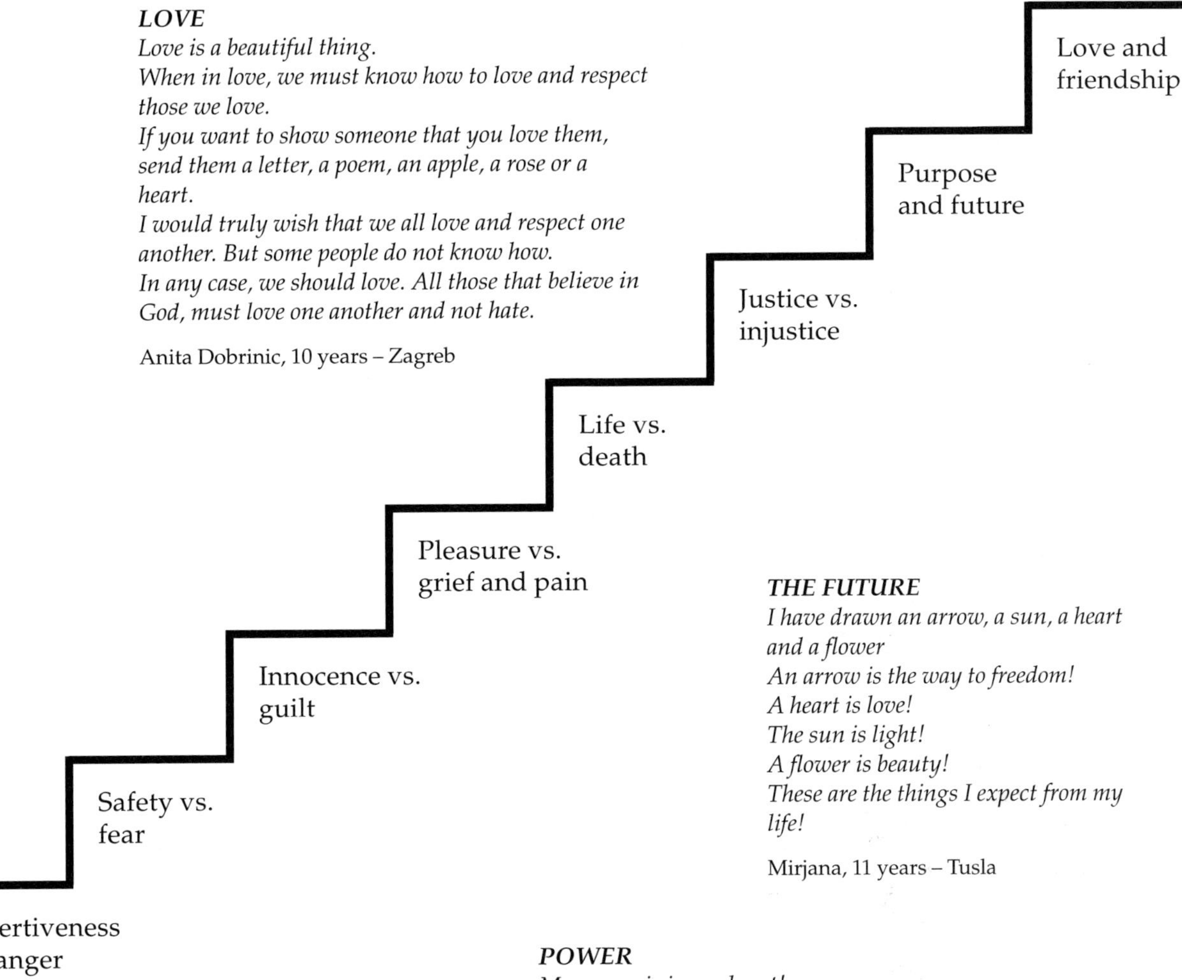

LOVE
Love is a beautiful thing.
When in love, we must know how to love and respect
those we love.
If you want to show someone that you love them,
send them a letter, a poem, an apple, a rose or a
heart.
I would truly wish that we all love and respect one
another. But some people do not know how.
In any case, we should love. All those that believe in
God, must love one another and not hate.

Anita Dobrinic, 10 years – Zagreb

THE FUTURE
I have drawn an arrow, a sun, a heart
and a flower
An arrow is the way to freedom!
A heart is love!
The sun is light!
A flower is beauty!
These are the things I expect from my
life!

Mirjana, 11 years – Tusla

POWER
My power is in my heart!

Gregor, 9 years – Sarajevo

POWER and HELPLESSNESS
My power is in Vukovar, in my home town.
My helplessness is in war.
My power is in faith.
My helplessness in the dark.
My power is in the light.
My helplessness is in fear.
Let there be an end to the war!

Marina, 11 years – Vukovar

To my grief I say: *I do not like you,*
You are dumb, dark and ugly,
Do not bother me, do not ever
come back again!

To my joy I say: *You are beautiful and good*
Follow me always
Stay with me every day
Grow, grow bigger and bigger!

Zvonko, 9 years – Zagreb

Appendix 3: Prvic refugee centre: information on family groups and individuals

Introduction

The following notes are based on informal discussions that took place during the pilot art therapy project with the psychologist and social worker at Prvic refugee centre in October and November 1994. Information is not comprehensive but contributed to ATI's understanding of the individuals and context in which the pilot projects took place. All names have been changed for the purposes of confidentiality.

Josipa (18), Emir (16), Ermin (15)

These three individuals are the youngest three children of a family of ten and come from a village in Bosnia near Zenica. All three arrived in Croatia three years earlier, before the war began, along with their elder sister (Alma) who was then 27 years old. Before arriving at Prvic they were together in another refugee camp in Rijeka called the Life Centre. When in Rijeka, Emir and Ermin became involved with a criminal circle and began to steal and commit minor offences for which they were caught (each time) and apprehended. Josipa was charged with three offences and Emir with seventeen. They were advised to leave Rijeka. Initially Alma came to Prvic with them but left very soon after.

Since then, Alma has had a baby and moved into a private house in Rijeka with a new boyfriend, leaving behind her brothers and sister. She has made empty promises which added to the siblings' sense of being left alone and neglected, and in need of guidance and love. Josipa, Emir and Ermin have very little contact with their parents, who remain in Bosnia, and seem to be waiting for some sort of direction with no plans for the future. Alma seems to have infrequent contact with her parents or siblings in Bosnia. In early October 1994 she had received news that two of their brothers (soldiers in Bosnia) were badly wounded.

Elma (mother) (30), Mari (10), Mario (8), Blazenka (4), Mirela (2)

This family are from Sarajevo. Elma was married at the age of seventeen but separated from her husband as a result of his alcoholism and violence. The latter led to him killing a man followed by his imprisonment, leaving the family threatened with blood revenge focusing on Mario. This, in conjunction with the war, led Elma to flee Sarajevo. Elma and her children have been refugees for two years, initially arriving in Trogir, near Split, where Elma met her present boyfriend (a Croatian soldier) They spent some time on Obanjan and managed to leave this island for Prvic. On Prvic, Elma was often absent for days at a time leaving Mari responsible for her brother and sisters. (In reality the children are taken care of by the other refugees.)

Refija (mother) (35), Hikmeta (7), Mihana (3), Mehmed (2)

The family came to Prvic from Sarajevo in July 1994, having lived in their apartment in a Muslim area throughout the war. Refija was a professor of Yugoslavian literature but also worked in administration as a secretary and accountant. In the last few years, she taught Croatian to UNPROFOR personnel. Her husband is a Serb who was in the Bosnian army and could therefore not leave Bosnia. Refija was forced to leave Sarajevo after their apartment was robbed and left empty. She had no job, was receiving threats from neighbours, with blood revenge directed at Mehmed. The family had wanted to go to Sweden but was refused entry by UNHCR as Sweden had stopped taking refugees. Refija recently had plans to go to Canada to stay with her cousin, and yet was reluctant to leave Croatia as it is closer to her husband. As a result of the war, until arriving on Prvic Mihana and Mehmed had lived entirely indoors and were therefore unused to physical activities and fresh air. They were also in poor health due to lack of food during the war. When they arrived on Prvic they were at first unable to digest the food and had gastro-intestinal problems. Refija was expecting another child.

Zlata (mother) (33), Ljuba (11), Zarina (6)

This family was originally from a Serb area in Tusla, now surrounded by Croatian borders. Zlata's husband, a Bosnian Serb in the Bosnian army, was unable to leave. Mersada is a Muslim. In April 1992, at the start of the war in Bosnia, their home was hit by a grenade. Zlata was a surgery nurse in the hospital. There were several reasons leading to her decision to leave Tusla: as a nurse, she had to go to work all the time and could not be with her children – adding to her stress; the wounds and traumatic situations she witnessed at the hospital and her personal wounds which she received when hit by shrapnel on the way to work in the head, arm and leg all led to a need for a safer environment. She arrived on Prvic determined to provide a future for her children.

Mina (mother) (17), Ivan (4 months)

Mina came from Herzegovina in 1990 and spent the four years, until she moved to Prvic, in Split with her parents who are Croatian. There, she attended adult education classes, specialising in cooking. She also met a Bosnian man ten years her senior and became pregnant. She was subsequently disowned by her parents. The boyfriend left her and went to Austria with his new girlfriend. As a result, Mina went to Prvic when Ivan was fourteen days old. Mina produced no milk of her own and there was shortage of milk and baby food in the centre. The Director did not see this as a priority and therefore the days would pass when the baby would drink only water with sugar. Eventually UNHCR obtained a large amount of milk powder. While on the island many of the refugees assisted in taking care of Ivan. At the end of October 1994, Mina was in the process of redeveloping a relationship with her parents and had left for Split to stay with them.

Gorana (23) and Goran (18)

Goran and Gorana are brother and sister and come from Banja-Luka. They left Bosnia for Croatia in 1991. Their parents, who are Croat and Muslim, remained in Banja-Luka which had become Serb-occupied. They had attempted in vain to exchange flats with a Serbian friend of theirs in Sarajevo as they did not want to leave Bosnia themselves. (They also have relatives in Norway.) Goran and Gorana hoped to return to Bosnia eventually. Initially, after leaving Bosnia, they stayed with an uncle in Sibenik and then moved on to Prvic. Their aunt is the head teacher of a school and organised for Goran to join it. Gorana worked at ODPR, the local office for refugees, but was made redundant. Following an argument over Goran's refusal to accept the authority of his uncle Goran left Sibenik and, finding himself homeless, joined the refugee centre on Prvic. Gorana followed a few weeks later. They had not seen their parents for three years, until the week ATI left Prvic, when the father managed to reach Sibenik to see his two children.

Sever (17) and Dejan (16)

These two brothers are from Sarajevo. Their mother had moved to Germany with her youngest son to join her husband there after spending 4 months on Prvic with her three sons. She now works as a house-cleaner. Prior to her leaving Bosnia, soldiers had broken into their house and she had to protect her sons by fighting back. She intended to return to Croatia in January 1995. Sever and Dejan decided to stay on Prvic in order to finish school, Dejan attending a school for drivers.

Elvis (17 years)

Elvis is the youngest of 11 brothers and sisters and the only member of his family at Prvic. He comes from somewhere in Bosnia. There is much confused information surrounding Elvis and his family history. It is suggested, for example, that his father was an alcoholic who killed his schizophrenic mother and then killed himself. Another version is that both his parents are still alive in Bosnia. It is understood that Elvis has lived in Croatia for several years, spending time in a school for children with 'mental disturbances' with one of his sisters. He also previously lived in a psychiatric department in Zagreb and at some stage attended a school for chefs. Before arriving on Prvic, Elvis lived for at least a year on Obanjan.

Elvis was initially placed in these homes as a result of extreme aggression and a threat towards himself and others. He had had a psychological assessment in Zagreb and was diagnosed as having mild brain damage. Since his arrival on Prvic, Elvis had displayed self-abusive behaviour and had threatened other residents. Although feared for his unpredictable behaviour he was also respected for his consideration of others.

Adisa (16)

Adisa was the only member of her family at Prvic. Her history is unclear as there is no official record of her past and it appears that some of the facts she reported are fabricated and inconsistent. It is understood that she is from Sarajevo. Adisa reported that her parents are divorced, were both alcoholics and violent towards her, once breaking her legs with a television. She also said that her parents are both dead, that her father was killed in the war and her mother died from a heart attack. She spoke about soldiers raping her and five friends and that her boyfriend was killed by a shell. Information from UNHCR suggested that Adisa was a prostitute in Sarajevo. On arrival on Prvic, Adisa displayed inconsistent behaviour but also an intelligence and physical maturity. She reported that UNHCR had arranged transit to Australia for her as soon as her visa is ready. She also expressed a desire to go to art school.

Azra (20)

Azra is from an undocumented town in Bosnia. Because she had only recently arrived on Prvic, the social workers knew little about her. She had only been on Prvic for three weeks on ATI's arrival. Azra had not seen her parents for three years and had moved from country to country alone, trying to find a place to settle. She lived for a while in Germany with her sister but had to return to Croatia to acquire a visa and appropriate papers. One of the other residents (Mina) is Azra's first cousin, although they had not met each other before. Azra had been married before the age of twenty and was now divorced, an experience that had caused her great pain and left her 'suspicious of relationships'. She arrived on Prvic ready to adapt to and accept the new challenges ahead of her.

Up-date on families
As communicated through letter on 25 April 1995 (by a volunteer working at the centre), it is understood that Zlata and family finally moved to Switzerland and Selver and Dejan have joined their family in Germany.

Appendix 4: ATI questionnaire – UNICEF's response

QUESTIONNAIRE

ART THERAPY INITIATIVE
FORMER YUGOSLAVIA 1994-96

<u>For: artists, art therapists, psychotherapists, mental health workers, project workers and researchers.</u>
<u>Re: Psychosocial Projects using art in the Former Yugoslavia.</u>

Throughout the war in the Former Yugoslavia art-making* has continued in a variety of settings in one form or another with children, young people and adults. This is taking place in kindergartens as a natural course of daily events with children, for example, or as an organised activity with the intention termed as 'therapeutic', occupational, educational, diagnostic or social.

While there seems to be a general understanding that art making has some value, ATI has found scarce information and no centralised documentation on this subject of art and art therapy in the Former Yugoslavia.   Integral to the research of ATI is the collating of such information so as to comprehensively understand what projects exist and in what capacity art is being used.   *We would therefore greatly appreciate your cooperation in filling out this questionnaire.*

Please fill out the questionnaire (circle appropriate answer) and return, if possible, by 3.6.96 to
ATI. 1/92 Kensington Church Street. London. W8 4BU

NAME: ....Rune Stuveland...

ORGANISATION: ...........UNICEF....B....and....H...................................

POSITION:...........Psycho-Social..Programme...Officer...........................

CONTACT ADDRESS: .....Fax 387 71 441 774..

TELEPHONE.: ....387 71 441 775...

1. Do you know of any *organised* art projects that exist or have existed

   in the Former Yugoslavia?   (Y)   N

   if yes:

       a) Where (e.g. town, city, country)..........Croatia, Slovenia, B and H.....................

       b) In what context (e.g. school, refugee camp).......Schools and Refugee camps....

       c) Run by whom (e.g. local, NGO)........Government, with UNICEF .... support........

       d) What form does/did it take: Please give details....Expressive drawings, puppetry, others

2. Do you know of any art therapy projects that exist or have existed in the F.Y.?   Y   N

   if yes:

       a) Where (e.g. town, city, country)...

       b) In what context (e.g. school, refugee camp)..

       c) Run by whom (e.g. local, NGO)...

       d) What form does/did it take: Please give details..

---

* Note: Art making is taken to mean any activity using the visual arts, music, drama or dance

3. Did you come across any *informal* art-making taking place in the Former Yugoslavia work?   Y   N

If yes:

    a) Where.....In war-affected areas..

    b) In what context........In shelters and collective centres etc............................

    c) What form did it take: Please give details.......During shelling: theatre groups, teachers and others would organize activities in shelters etc.....................................

4. Have you come across any written documentation on art or art therapy in this context?   Y   N

If yes

    a) Could you name it..........ARPAD BARATH / UNICEF....................................

    b) Is it available to the public.......YES............... If yes, where.......AUTHOR via UNICEF...

5. ATI has found that the Profession of Art Therapy is unfamiliar to most people. It would be useful to learn how you understand art therapy

6. Any other information that you think may be useful in this context

7. Any questions you would like to ask ATI

Would be interested in feedback - maybe make a conference on art therapy in war?

We would like to thank you for you co-operation in filling out this questionnaire and intend to include the results in our research document in the coming months.

If you are interested in receiving further information on art therapy or ATI reasearch findings

please tick the box   ☒

Debra Kalmanowitz
Bobby Lloyd
The Art Therapy Initiative - Former Yugoslavia 1994-96
May 1996

Appendix 5: The Art Works Trust: 'The need'

The following information was provided by The Art Works Trust:
'A 1994 survey by Dr Beverley Killian (Department of Psychology, University of Natal, Pietermaritzburg) showed that in KwaZulu–Natal:

- 84% of black children in urban areas suffered from symptoms of Post-Traumatic Stress Disorder or major depression.
- 33% had psychological symptoms serious enough to warrant clinical diagnosis.
- 33% of pre-school children drew pictures of violence in progress.

A significant number of children in this study wished to die.

A survey with primary school children found that:

- 2.6% had killed someone
- 3.6% had participated in a killing
- 27% had seen someone being killed (47% in high school)
- 20% had had their homes burned or attacked
- 25% of girls and 11% of boys were sexually abused

In much of KwaZulu–Natal there is an intermittent ongoing civil war. Part of the legacy of apartheid, its roots are in poverty, overcrowding, competition for limited jobs and resources, political rivalry. Crime – and increasingly – drug trafficking play a part. A generation has grown up accepting as the norm unacceptable levels of violence. The situation needs addressing urgently if the cycle of violence is to be broken.

It is felt that training and understanding of the skills and insights of art therapy could help those working in this field.'

Appendix 6: Workplaces of workshop participants in KwaZulu–Natal

Medical Foundation for the Care of Victims
Counsellor

School Psychological Services
Educational psychologist

KwaZulu–Natal Survivors of Violence
Clinical psychologist

Children and Violence in South Africa
Nurse

Children and Violence in South Africa
Psychiatric nurse

Natal Society of Arts Outreach Programme
Artist

Claremont
Teacher/counsellor

Durban
Clinical psychologist

University of Natal Department of Psychology
Clinical psychologist

Appendix 7: Workshop Questionnaire

Used at the start of the art therapy workshops in KwaZulu–Natal:

We would be grateful if you would fill in this short questionnaire and hand it to either Debra or Bobby at the end of the first day.

1. What were your initial reasons for joining the workshop?

2. What do you wish to take with you after the four weeks?

3. Where do you hope the workshop will lead you?

4. Any other comments or thoughts at this stage.

Appendix 8: Workshop evaluation form

1. Please give an overall evaluation of the course.

2. Which part of the course did you find the most useful?

3. Which part did you find the least relevant to you?

4. Do you have any other suggestions or thoughts at this stage?

5. On a scale of 0–5 where 0 is the lowest and 5 is the highest, please rate the various components of the workshop:

1. Open art therapy studios   0   1   2   3   4   5
2. Open studios (Saturdays)
3. Interactive art therapy group
4. Materials workshop
5. Theme workshop
6. Materials discussion
7. Case conference
8. Seminar
9. Overall

Appendix 9: Course programme evaluation table

Participant:	A	B	C	D	E	F	G	H	I
Open art therapy studio	4	5	4	5	5	4	5	5	5
Open studios (Saturday)	4	3	3	3	5	3	4	4	5
Interactive art therapy group	5	5	5	5	5	4	5	5	5
Materials workshop	3	3	4	4	5	4	5	5	5
Theme workshop	3	4	3	4	3	3	5	4	4
Case conference	2	5	5	4	2	3	5	5	5
Seminar	2	5	4	3	3–5	3	5	5	5
Overall	5	5	5	5	5	4	5	5	5

On a scale of 0–5 where 0 is the lowest and 5 is the highest, participants were asked to rate the various components of the workshop. The average overall score was 4.9.